Engineers and Communities

Engineers and Communities

Transforming Sanitation in Contemporary Brazil

Earthea Nance

LEXINGTON BOOKS
Lanham • Boulder • New York • Toronto • Plymouth, UK

Published by Lexington Books
A wholly owned subsidiary of The Rowman & Littlefield Publishing Group, Inc.
4501 Forbes Boulevard, Suite 200, Lanham, Maryland 20706
www.rowman.com

10 Thornbury Road, Plymouth PL6 7PP, United Kingdom

British Library Cataloguing in Publication Information Available

Library of Congress Cataloging-in-Publication Data Available

978-0-7391-2681-3 (cloth : alk. paper)
978-0-7391-7928-4 (electronic)

™ The paper used in this publication meets the minimum requirements of American National Standard for Information Sciences—Permanence of Paper for Printed Library Materials, ANSI/NISO Z39.48-1992.

Printed in the United States of America

To my beloved children, Ntwari and Mutoni

Contents

Preface

My first visit to Brazil was in 1992, the same year as the first Rio Earth Summit, and everyone was talking about sustainability. I was there as a graduate student seeking a research project and practicing my very new Portuguese language skills. That summer I traveled through most of the country, meeting with dozens of environmental professionals in the states of Rio de Janeiro, São Paulo, Brasília, Bahia, Amazonas, and Paraná. Of the many pressing environmental issues in Brazil that had attracted international attention (such as deforestation of the Amazon rainforest, expansion of hydroelectric power, protection of biodiversity, and conservation of the Pantanal wetlands), I wanted to find out which environmental issues were of most concern to Brazilians. During these conversations I learned about an emerging new technology called *condominial* sewerage. It was still brand new. Success was not assured. But, unanimously, each expert I spoke with thought the new approach was promising because it might improve the quality of life for the majority of people in Brazil, and it was therefore deserving of study.

I wrote this book to gain a deeper understanding of how a pioneering group of Brazilian engineers was able to transform their sanitation sector to make it more inclusive. In harmony with the sustainability perspective, *Engineers and Communities* tackles this question by integrating engineering and social science ways of knowing. The theories and methods in this book draw from civil and environmental engineering, anthropology, area studies (Latin America), science and technology studies, and urban development studies. This approach parallels my personal journey from practicing engineer to interdisciplinary scholar. It is my hope that *Engineers and Communities* will inspire other scholars and practitioners who are interested in integrating their knowledge. But even more, I hope this book expands interest in the potential of the participatory sanitation paradigm to create space for innovations that expand access to basic urban services.

My efforts to write this book benefitted from the support of several generous institutions. I am grateful to Massachusetts Institute of Technology for providing me with a full year of support to write the draft manuscript and to conduct the second phase of fieldwork in Brazil. This book builds upon my graduate student research, and I am grateful for the generous support I received from Stanford University which provided several travel and writing grants, from the World Bank that provided two internships in its water and sanitation division, and from the Buck Foundation that provided a full year of support to conduct the first phase of fieldwork in Brazil. Access to the raw data that was generated by this research is available at Stanford University Library (UMI No. 3128354).

Acknowledgments

I am thankful for the many friends, colleagues, and mentors who assisted me over the years as I wrote this book. I especially want to thank Judith Tendler, Leonard Ortolano, Renia Ehrenfeucht, and Sybil Ohagwu. And to my family, who remained supportive even when this project took me away from them, I am forever grateful.

Chapter 1
The Promise and Failure of Development

In the 1990s, the major international development agencies—including the U.S. Agency for International Development, the United Nations, and the World Bank—made a fundamental shift toward a new approach to ending global poverty.[1] The new approach was to directly involve people in the planning and implementation of infrastructure services, especially in local water and sanitation projects, which were considered an important component of human and economic development. It was thought that people's direct involvement in infrastructure projects would bring crucial services to population groups that had been excluded from the promise of development. The new approach became known by terms such as "bottom-up," "grassroots," or "participatory" development. One of the most significant experiments in participatory development has been taking place in Brazil's water and sanitation sector since the early 1980s. This book describes and evaluates this experience and seeks to understand how a participatory approach to sanitation evolved in Brazil. The Brazilian case offers important lessons for scholars and practitioners of development, and sheds light on a fundamental question: can the promise of participatory development be realized?

The Global Water and Sanitation Problem

The failure of development is inequity—inequity that is tolerated at extreme levels. Nowhere is this inequity more visible than in the global water and sanitation sector, where the significance of the problem is clear and easy to summarize. According to the United Nations, over 1.2 billion people lacked clean water and over 2.4 billion people lacked adequate sanitation at the beginning of the millennium.[2] The great majority of people without these services live in developing countries of the Global South, also known as the majority world on the basis of its far greater population.[3] Reducing these numbers by half by the year 2015 is one of eight Millennium Development Goals established by world leaders in September 2000 at the UN Millennium Summit.

Further illustrating the magnitude of the sanitation problem for the majority world are two interrelated trends: urbanization and sanitation-related disease. Increasingly, the Earth's human population is urbanized. In 2001, 47 percent of the planet's human population lived in cities, and this percentage is expected to increase to 60 percent by 2030.[4] A significant number of people also endure the health consequences of inadequate sanitation. The World Health Organization (WHO) estimates that 40 percent of the global population was living without sewage disposal facilities in 2000.[5] Inadequate sanitation is linked to endemic diseases such as intestinal parasitic infections, schistosomiasis, and diarrheal diseases that kill over 2.2 million people per year worldwide, mostly children under five years of age.[6] The majority of those affected by endemic sanitation-related diseases are poverty-stricken and low income people who live in the Global South. In contrast, epidemic sanitation-related diseases such as cholera and typhoid can affect the general population (although everyone is not equally susceptible).

These mind-numbing statistics illustrate the widening gap between rich and poor even in newly-industrializing countries that have realized at least some of the promise of development, of which Brazil is a good example. In 1999, the Pan American Health Organization (PAHO) estimated that 81.7 percent of the Brazilian population resided in urban areas, making Brazil one of the most urbanized countries in the world.[7] Moreover, just over 50 percent of urban households in Brazil were connected to sewers in 2001.[8] As a consequence, diarrheal disease was among the main causes of mortality and morbidity in Brazilian children under five years of age.[9] In Brazil and elsewhere, the sanitation crisis is disproportionately endured by people who are disenfranchised from formal service delivery systems. If they have service at all, it is typically an onsite system such as a latrine, leach pit, cesspool, or septic tank—the sanitation systems most often used by people living in urban poverty.

Continued reliance on these kinds of systems is becoming increasingly infeasible. Onsite sanitation systems can provide a safe means of waste disposal only up to a certain point. At low and medium population densities (measured as number of people per hectare), onsite sanitation systems are a feasible solution for reducing the risk of sanitation-related disease in rural and urban areas.[10] But at the high population densities typical of today's cities, onsite systems can actually provoke sanitation-related disease by permanently contaminating the surrounding soils and groundwater. As population densities increase around the world, cities have to question the long-term feasibility of onsite sanitation and consider transitioning to sewerage systems for public health reasons.[11]

Sewerage is a "system of pipes for wastewater collection and removal" commonly referred to as a sewer; while *sanitation* refers more broadly to "services or systems of collection, transportation, treatment, and sanitary disposal of wastewater, excreta, or other waste."[12] Several features characterize the conventional sewer system. Houses with a conventional sewer system usually face the street and are laid out regularly on city blocks. Houses are connected individually to a sewer pipe located in the street, and streets are paved and of ample width to allow vehicular access by personnel who maintain the sewer lines. Relatively large-diameter sewer pipes are installed at conservative (i.e., relatively steep) design slopes and depths. Expensive equipment and materials must be available to construct and maintain conventional sewer systems. Finally, there must be a suitable destination to receive the collected sewage, such as a well-operated wastewater treatment plant, so that the ecological carrying capacity of surrounding water bodies is not exceeded.

Many cities in the Global South, including Brazilian cities, have not yet developed the physical or financial capacity to support the above-described "conventional" sewerage system for the entire population.[13] As a consequence, conventional sewers in Brazil mainly serve more affluent neighborhoods that have the conditions to receive and afford conventional sewer systems,[14] while disenfranchised neighborhoods primarily use onsite systems or no formal system at all—not by choice but by default. The resulting inequity has been allowed to persist. The Brazilian Census Bureau (IBGE) reported that, in 2001, 86 percent of households with incomes of five or more minimum salaries per capita had adequate sanitation.[15] Conversely, only 38 percent of households in extreme poverty (i.e., with incomes of 0.5 or less minimum salaries per capita) had adequate sanitation. Given that 62 percent of Brazilian workers earned only two minimum salaries or less in the early 2000s,[16] solving the sanitation problem means addressing the physical, financial, and social limitations faced by the majority of the population.

Why Sanitation Services Fail the Urban Poor

One of the first lessons to learn from the Global South's experience is that conventional sewer systems cannot address the sanitation needs of the majority world because of its different physical, financial, and social circumstances. The physical circumstances of most unsewered residential neighborhoods give rise to a series of technical challenges, many of which cannot be resolved using conventional sewer technology. As in most developing and newly-industrializing countries, the majority of urban homes in Brazil were constructed without underground sewer infrastructure such as pipes, manholes, and pump stations. In some instances, homes were constructed below the elevation of the street, in flood plains, or in other poorly drained areas, which makes sewage collection more technically challenging and which may require the provision of pavement and drainage in addition to a sewer system. Without careful engineering or the provision of complementary infrastructure such as pavement and drainage, sewer systems in poorly drained areas will not function effectively.

Some urban residents do not have adequate access to water or bathrooms in or near the home, so the provision of a sewer system to these households must be accompanied by the provision of water supply systems and sanitation facilities, which increases the scope and cost of any proposed sewer project. If water is only supplied a few days per week rather than daily (which is the case in many poor and low income urban Brazilian neighborhoods), and if bathrooms are not plumbed or connected to the sewer, then the operational benefits of a proposed sewer system—in terms of improved public health and environmental quality—cannot be realized. Many urban neighborhoods are characterized by irregular housing layouts, indistinct blocks, narrow unpaved pathways instead of streets, and a lack of public rights-of-way. These characteristics impede the installation of conventional sewer systems, and preclude access by conventional sewer construction equipment and sewer maintenance trucks. In these situations, conventional sewers are either never constructed or, if constructed, they function poorly because they cannot be properly maintained.

In most developing countries, the financial incentives for market-run conventional sewer service have been too low to stimulate large-scale private investment. Likewise, the financial costs of state-run conventional sewer service have been too high to be sustained.[17] For these reasons, private firms have had little incentive to enter into markets for public goods like sewer systems, and in Brazil no one has required them to do so. The high capital and maintenance costs of conventional sewage collection and treatment systems pose another challenge. Conventional sewers are expensive as a result of high design standards promoted by the engineering and urban planning professions, ostensibly to protect public health. Average capital costs for conventional sewers in developing countries are in the neighborhood of US$650 per connection; however, using simplified sewers can result in an average savings of 44 percent.[18] Conventional sewer costs in Brazil range from approximately $200 per capita (in 1992 U.S. dollars) for sewers alone to approximately $1000 per capita for conventional sewers plus treatment.[19] Historically, Brazilian agencies responsible for water and sanitation have had limited public resources available for the construction of new sewer infrastructure, and elected leaders have not been willing or able to address this problem. The majority of Brazil's population cannot afford the fees associated with conventional sewer service, and when fees are heavily subsidized the financial shortfall to water and sanitation agencies can ultimately contribute to inadequate public investment in sewer system expansion, sewage treatment, and sewer system maintenance. The result is a downward cycle of underdevelopment in the sector, not only in Brazil but in most countries of the Global South.

For many reasons, sewer projects must often be accompanied by educational and promotional campaigns to change the habit patterns of potential users.[20] Residents may not be educated about the relationship between sewer systems and disease.[21] Unless people have this knowledge, it is generally difficult to stimulate public demand for sewer infrastructure. Residents may not express demand for sanitary sewers until their demands for other higher-priority services (e.g., land tenure, electricity, and water) have been satisfied.[22] Demand for sanitary sewers tends to increase as urban population densities increase, as water supplies increase, and as incomes increase.[23] Some residents may not want to interact with government officials out of fear of eviction, mistrust, or apathy resulting from previous project failures and a history of broken promises.[24] Residents may also believe that a new system will be too expensive or that user fees will change each time a new official is elected,[25] so they may not express demand for a system. As long as each household finds an individual disposal solution, community-level health and environmental problems may have to reach crisis levels before they are widely perceived, and even then the demand for sanitation may be based on desires for privacy and convenience rather than public or personal health.

The technical, financial, and social dimensions of sanitation just described are reflected in three general outcomes that can be observed in Brazil and many other countries of the Global South: 1) typically low rates of sewer coverage (i.e., the percent of population with access to sanitary sewers), 2) poorly performing sewer systems in general (although this is rarely measured), and 3) a geographic patchwork of sewer service sharply differentiated by income, with affluent areas receiving the limited services that are available and lower income areas remaining unserved (i.e., disenfranchised from the service delivery network) and relying on individual onsite solutions. The inability of either markets or states to ensure peoples' rights to basic life-support services, including basic sanitation, threatens living conditions, public health, and environmental quality in Brazil and elsewhere. And the increasing rate of urbanization only exacerbates these problems in areas that still rely on onsite systems. All sanitation-related diseases are preventable, yet they kill millions of people per year.

Given this array of obstacles, the sanitation problem is not likely to be solved merely by expanding conventional sewers to population groups that are disenfranchised under the current state of affairs. A promising solution to the complexities of the sanitation problem emerged in Brazil in the early 1980s. The new approach involved transitioning from a conventional approach to an approach based on appropriate technology and participation that could overcome technical, financial, and social constraints at the neighborhood level. The remainder of this book describes the emergence and evolution of Brazil's new approach to sanitation and critically interprets this experience in light of current thinking about pro-poor approaches to development.

Why Brazil Is a Critical Case

Historical inequity in the distribution of water and sanitation services in Brazil is a good example of social exclusion. The great majority of Brazil's population was excluded from access to these important services, making Brazil a critical case for understanding the effectiveness of specific reforms designed to overcome social exclusion in the water and sanitation sector. Brazil's reforms included a transformation of state-society relations at the national level via democratization and decentralization, and a significant increase in the agency of individuals at the local level through a multitude of participatory processes and appropriate technologies. During Brazil's transition to democracy (1984–1995), municipalities gained access to federal funding and sought to expand access to public services such as water and sanitation. Corresponding with this decentralization of funding, the prevailing model for delivering basic infrastructure services changed from a conventional approach to a participatory approach characterized by the involvement of citizens in public policy making and public service delivery. In the water and sanitation sector, the new approach employed lower cost technology and community participation in planning and implementation. The change was significant because it increased local power in the water and sanitation sector and promised to extend services to vast numbers of unserved citizens. Brazil appears to have institutionalized the key elements—decentralized governance, community participation, and appropriate technology—for extending water and sanitation service to all neighborhoods. Because of these multiple advantages, many observers in the early 1980s predicted great achievements in Brazil's water and sanitation sector. This promise was further solidified with the advent of participatory budgeting in the early 1990s.

Brazil is also a critical case for examining whether the theories of participatory democracy and participatory development hold up in practice. Scholars and practitioners have identified citizen participation as one of the keys to success in delivering infrastructure services in developing countries.[26] Despite widespread acceptance of the value of participation, there are still significant gaps in knowledge. The lack of information about how people participate in local projects and the lack of critical evaluation of the impact of their participation are obstacles to understanding how to extend the promise of development without continued exclusion. Previous research concludes that people participate very differently in different cities and neighborhoods, and that understanding the local context is crucial for discerning what works in the delivery of basic sanitation services.[27] Brazil's unique experience with community participation on a large scale across diverse urban settings is worthy of in-depth study. The enormous challenge of extending basic infrastructure services to people around the world makes understanding Brazil's experience critical for the 2.4 billion people who still lack basic sanitation services and for an untold number whose systems are inappropriate or dysfunctional.

Methodology

There is little theory to guide one through the myriad dilemmas that present themselves in the course of conducting interdisciplinary cross-cultural research about the concerns of marginalized people of the world. In this section, I present the principles, sources, and methods that governed my research about Brazil's attempt to overcome social exclusion in its distribution of basic infrastructure services. Among the most salient concerns of my research were the possibilities for cultural misinterpretation and the perception and use of power. I used the following guiding principles to address these concerns: 1) the application of locally relevant and detailed conceptual frames rather than the imposition of general purpose frames derived from other contexts; 2) the use of ethnographic case study analysis nested across spatial scales (e.g., project, neighborhood, city, and regional scales); 3) the use of iteration as a methodology (i.e., re-measuring the same variable in different ways); and 4) the incorporation of multiple voices as the only defensible approach for research that does not merely reproduce the thoughts and judgments of those in power. As a consequence, the book departs significantly from mainstream methods used in the water and sanitation sector and draws equally from engineering, the social sciences, and science and technology studies. The result is simultaneously a description, an evaluation, and a critique of Brazil's experience.

The evidence and analyses presented in the book are based on four fundamental methodologies. First is a comprehensive literature review of mainstream accounts of participatory development (chapter 1), and a description of specific water and sanitation reforms associated with Brazil's period of democratization (chapter 2). The second methodology is a comparative analysis of condominial sewerage in two Brazilian cities, which involved over a year of fieldwork (chapters 3, 4, and 5). Third is a comparative theory-building case study of project performance for seven condominial sewer projects, resulting in an explanatory framework based on project coalitions (chapter 6). Fourth is a content analysis of oral and written texts presented by engineers and officials who created and disseminated the paradigm of participatory sanitation from city to city in Brazil, contrasted with what was learned in previous chapters about actual implementation experiences (chapter 7).

In all, I conducted semi-structured interviews with 297 randomly selected households in seven Brazilian neighborhoods,[28] I conducted semi-structured interviews with twenty-five practitioners and officials from seven implementing agencies; and I held focus groups with residents and community leaders in several neighborhoods. I also conducted informal interviews with over seventy-five project managers, engineers, social scientists, and maintenance staff of the implementing agencies; with elected officials and appointed agency directors involved in planning and funding the case study projects; with community leaders and residents; and with other relevant personnel such as selected employees of consulting firms and construction companies who worked as contractors for the implementing agencies, as well as sanitation specialists from Brazil, the World Bank, and elsewhere. In addition to the interviews and focus groups, I drew from multiple sources of information, including direct observations, project inspections, neighborhood transect walks, document reviews, and archival sources.

A Theoretical History of Development Accounts

In their sweeping review of the theoretical history of development, Pritchett and Woolcock conclude that there is no consensus for action, that there is no basis for knowing what will work to improve service delivery in any particular development sector or locale, and that there are no conditions for replicating successful development outcomes.[29] They argue that the problem lies in seeking a single solution to development and that reliance on an all-purpose account of development has led to theoretical confusion and objective failure regardless of which account was adopted. Pritchett and Woolcock elegantly demonstrate that our inability to establish useful accounts of development practice is significant and has resulted in gross failure. Below I describe this situation from my own perspective. In my view, two fundamental views of development are most relevant: the universalist account and the relativist account.

The Post-World War II Universalist Account of Development

The first wave of development discourse that emerged after World War II (1940s–1960s) was presented within a universalizing ontology (or knowledge order). Universalizing (also called essentializing, generalizing, or totalizing) knowledge is usually sustained by the creation of ontological divides.[30] For example, the universalist account viewed expert knowledge as right/good/legitimate and lay knowledge as wrong/bad/irrelevant to the Development project,[31] while simultaneously denying the construction of this divide. Within a universalist worldview, development was progress and progress was always good, so it followed that "undeveloped" people needed development. This "world-ordering knowledge"[32] was considered to be a self-evident fact that was not subject to discussion or debate, and so few of the disciplines problematized development itself.[33] A less abstract restatement of the universalist view of development, using sanitation development as an example, would be something like the following.

> Sanitary conditions in much of the Third World are at the levels of Europe in the mid-1800s, with the attendant endemic water and sanitation-related diseases (e.g., cholera, typhoid, dysentery, etc.). Basic sanitation technologies that have existed for over 100 years have still not reached underdeveloped areas. The solution to the lack of development already exists: we who have the know-how must transfer our technology to countries in need and teach them how to use it. Bringing development to people living in poverty is the right thing to do.

The above account is based on the assumption that so-called "Third World" people—a now obsolete term that emerged simultaneously with the first wave of post-World War II development discourse—needed development and that First World people were in a position to define and deliver that development. Within the universalist account, a "bad" development condition justified the imposition of a knowledge order that was assumed to contain no social content and therefore was not subject to inspection. Conventional water and sanitation development falls within this universalist knowledge order.

Participatory Development: A Post-1970s Relativist Response

Relativist critiques of the universalist view of development saw universalism as a construct of domination, as the imposition of a singular solution that marginalized some individuals for an imagined greater good. Participatory approaches to development that valued the needs of communities over and above universal approaches thus emerged in second wave accounts of development (i.e., 1970s–1990s). Relativists saw the universalist view not as universally true but as culturally situated. This approach established a knowledge order in which local community decisions were preferable, more appropriate, and necessary to counter First World attempts to use its dominant position to impose a set of external standards that might be inappropriate.[34] Within the relativist view, universal knowledge was "wrong" because it lacked social content, thereby justifying the imposition of a pure, local, social order. An example of the relativist view of development, again with sanitation as the example, would be something like the following.

> Development is not a simple matter of experts transferring pre-existing solutions from developed countries to underdeveloped countries. People need to participate in the sanitation systems that are being extended to them, and their involvement should include not only education about the value of sanitation. Techniques like Participatory Rural Appraisal (and its urban variants) allow people to take part in sanitation project decision-making through all phases of the project cycle. Moreover, new sanitation technologies need to be offered that are appropriate to local conditions. A bottom-up, people-centered approach to development will be more successful than the top-down development approaches of the past.

Although all of the participation literature does not say the same thing, the central proposition of the participatory development literature was that better participation would lead to better development outcomes.[35] A number of theoretical arguments were put forward in support of this proposition during the second wave of development accounts, including post-colonial, neoliberal, marginality, democratization, governance and, more recently, sustainability frameworks. The post-colonial framework viewed participation as a way to counter the legacy of colonial institutions.[36] The neoliberal perspective valued participation as a way to reveal people's willingness to pay, to facilitate "getting the prices right" and to help match demand with supply.[37] In marginality theory, people who were marginalized by development were perceived as having certain traits and deficits, such as a lack of education, lack of cultural capital, etc., and participation was viewed as a way to overcome these deficits.[38] The democratization framework viewed participation as a way to expand people's citizenship rights.[39] In recognition of the failure of top-down approaches, theories of bureaucracy and governance emerged in support of bottom-up, participatory approaches to development.[40] And finally, sustainable development frameworks advanced participation as a way to change people's consumptive and polluting behaviors.[41] All of these epistemological frameworks supported a positive attitude toward participatory development; however, none of these accounts could be characterized as critical and all relied on inherited universalist constructs such as "First" and "Third" world, "poverty," and most of all "development."[42]

Deconstructing Participatory Development

While participatory development can be broadly characterized as a relativist critique of the earlier universalist development account, this stance results in an uncomfortable asymmetry: development for the minority world (e.g., conventional forms of infrastructure services implemented for middle- and upper-income beneficiaries in the Global North and the Global South), and *participatory* development for the majority world (e.g., alternative forms of infrastructure services implemented almost exclusively for poor and low income people in the Global South).[43] The following section deconstructs participatory development along three main lines of critique: bias, dominance, and inequity.

Second wave accounts of participatory development were generally biased because they were presented, discussed, and recommended as if participation were universally applicable and neutral[44] and as if Western forms of development were the norm. The participatory development literature was also biased toward a hopeful emphasis on the possibilities for empowerment. Instead of showcasing the full range of competing narratives, the participatory development literature highlighted only a single narrative. In that narrative, participatory development promised to enhance voice and accountability between users and authorities and to reveal local knowledge and demand. Participatory development was thought to impart a sense of empowerment and ownership, to increase community capacity, and to diversify technology options to meet local needs and gain cultural acceptance. In other words, participation was always viewed as good.

Furthermore, dominant forms of participatory development were often sponsored by the powerful (such as by the World Bank), but forms of participation that emerged from the grassroots (such as organized resistance) were unwanted by those in power. Another sign of dominance was the use of participatory development as a mechanism for appropriating unpaid labor. Participatory development programs often emphasized labor-intensive activities and direct involvement over indirect participation, effective representation, and state action.

Although participatory development was presented and used as a unifying, equalizing concept, it was in practice used to both unify and divide, to open up and to shut down political discussion, to include and to exclude people from development. Not widely discussed in the literature was the separate-but-so-called-equal nature of participatory development. In this sense, participatory development was a type of ethnodevelopment, a site of othering that established a different set of rules for a specific segment of the population, while development (unqualified) was intended for everyone else. Like the labeling of various ethnoknowledges (e.g., ethnomathematics, ethnohistory, ethnoreligion, ethnomusicology, etc.) that signified which knowledges were considered ancient, non-Western, or unscientific, the term "participatory development" created and solidified inequality and otherness by naturalizing class difference and marginality.

Further aspects of bias, dominance, and inequity are evident in the conceptualization of participation along a single axis. Arnstein's (1969) axis, called a "ladder of participation," ordered participation along a scale from Manipulation (minimum citizen power and maximum state control) to Citizen Control (maximum citizen power and autonomy from the state).[45] This was a generalized account of where power resided, based on the assumption that pre-existing states of power within individuals or groups corresponded with various levels of participation with the state, and that maximum autonomy from the state was a universal goal. But organized poor people seeking autonomy from the state (i.e., Citizen Control) are generally considered dangerous rather than ideal expressions of empowered participation; and because of this bias poor people could not actualize themselves by faithfully climbing their way up Arnstein's ladder of participation. On the other hand, non-poor groups who were assumed to hold greater levels of power and autonomy could more often rely on the state to serve their infrastructure needs without needing to participate. Each of these scenarios appears to contradict the implied continuity of the axis. The Arnstein ladder attempted to generalize static conditions of decision authority held by various groups (represented by their degree of participation) but was discontinuous in practice for any particular group, so it was an axis only in an abstract, Cartesian sense. It was not intended to describe actual movement or empowerment, nor did movement up the axis necessarily indicate better outcomes or even greater power.

Choguill's (1996) participation axis attempted to address the discontinuities of the Arnstein axis by recognizing the fact that poverty-stricken people in developing countries were neglected by the state (hence their poverty), and their participation was an attempt to resolve this neglect rather than to gain Citizen Control.[46] The Choguill axis varied from Self Management (citizen autonomy and agency neglect) to Empowerment (full status as a client or beneficiary of the state). This was a generalized account of subjecthood, which assumed that neglected groups wanted to become enfranchised by moving up Choguill's ladder of participation and that maximum enfranchisement was the ideal expression of empowered participation. But would non-poor groups seeking autonomy from the state become empowered at the top of the Choguill ladder (i.e., when the state had maximum control)? Likely not. The Choguill axis theorized continuous empowerment for a particular group, but this came at the expense of generalizing a single path of empowerment that did not apply to all groups.

Both the Arnstein and Choguill axes of participation in development were internally coherent yet incompatible when applied to real circumstances and actual groups, raising questions about the preconceived expected benefits of participation. Each axis was an attempt to describe a state of affairs that could not be understood with only a single axis of action; each assumed that power pre-existed the performance of participation (and that participation was therefore a representation of power); and each evoked an idealized expression of empowered participation.

The foregoing deconstruction of participatory development exposes the bias, dominance, and inequity of mainstream relativist accounts. While participatory development emerged in reaction to prior universalist accounts of development, it is nevertheless conceived as universally applicable and universally good, rendering it biased. The use of participatory development as a tool for empowerment is repeatedly affirmed even as its use as a dominating process is denied. And rather than posing a direct challenge to inequities, participatory development often naturalizes pre-existing structural inequities. It is customary to speak of participatory development in terms of generalized accounts rather than practice-based accounts. By defining from the top down the acceptable forms, paths, and goals of participation, the diversity of participatory acts in particular places and times is made to look more ordered and science-like, and therefore superior to "mere" social phenomena which in a universalist mind-set are considered inferior. Participatory development discourse has become fixed, unable to explain failure, offer real critique, or distinguish among effective and ineffective forms of participation, even with the benefit of ladders of participation. These misgivings about participatory development expose its status as a fundamentally contested concept.[47]

Actors, Action, and the Post-Structural Perspective

Having come through a first wave in which post-World War II accounts of development were primarily based on universalist perspectives, and then through a second wave characterized by post-1970 relativist critiques of universalist development based on the notion of participatory development, we are now in a third wave of understanding. In rethinking development, it is instructive to recognize that the universalist and relativist frameworks were in fact a duality of a single underlying ontological structure. Both the universalist and relativist frameworks relied on an agreed upon divide between the scientific and the social, between content and context, subject and object, First World and Third World. This structural condition of modern thought is known by various names, such as foundationism[48] or the Modern Constitution.[49] Healy explained the notion of the Modern Constitution as follows:

> Natural science equips us with explanations centring on an 'external' material reality while the social sciences identify concerns centring upon the views, practices, behaviours and effects of social actors and institutions, but our capacity to grasp the intermeshing of the two remains poor. This rigid distinction between non-human material and human socio-cultural domains endures because it is a foundational feature of Western metaphysics, deriving from Cartesian mind/body dualism but with sources reaching back to at least Plato (e.g., see Latour, 1999, chs. 7 and 8). (Stephen Healy, 2005, 2)

Both universalism and relativism required the maintenance (in thought and in discourse) of divides to separate what were believed to be pure objects and pure subjects, pure physical science and pure social science. Both universalism and relativism required belief in generalization, albeit within different prescribed disciplines separated by solid divides. Latour, Mol, and others have written extensively on the idea that people and things are not pure subjects and objects in practice (i.e., in "action"); rather, they are subjectified and objectified in discourse. These authors have observed that in action nothing is pure; on the contrary, everything is mixed, interrelated, hybrid; and that neither science-based knowledge nor social-based knowledge is pure. Despite claims to the contrary, universalism does not represent one singular thing, and relativism does not represent a plurality of discrete things. The existence of any discrete thing depends on the maintenance of structural boundaries that allow it to exist discretely. In action, things are neither fact nor fiction, neither purely discursive nor purely real, but a combination of each holding a relative state of existence.[50] This is the position from which this book will analyze participatory development.

If one recognizes that objectivity requires a discursive element; or, in Latour's view, if facts are facts *because* they are made; and if making objects requires the construction of ontological dichotomies (e.g., material versus social), then it becomes possible to consider participatory development as action leading to co-produced urban services, for example, and discourse about co-produced urban services. It also becomes possible to consider that the bias of participatory development—the notion that participation is always beneficial—has a purpose in discourse whether or not it is true in action. By questioning what divides were constructed in the making of participatory development and by pondering how those divides might be transformed, it is possible to restore symmetry. An actor-oriented account of participatory development opens up the possibility of new ways of understanding development that are not bound by the structural divides of universalism and relativism.

Scholars and practitioners of development are beginning to intuit the ideas so elegantly stated by post-structural thinkers. Those working from within a discipline, any discipline, no longer believe their discipline has a lock on truth. More and more scholars are reaching across the imagined divide between the scientific and the social in search of better ways of knowing the world. Even the most powerful organizations, such as the U.S. National Science Foundation, have begun encouraging and funding multi- and inter-disciplinary research. But despite having taken the first steps into a third wave of thinking about development (which occurred primarily in the 2000s when open critique of participatory development surfaced), most of the concepts and frameworks from the first and second waves are still in active use. The biases and inequities of participatory development, summarized previously, are now broadly felt and seen, but they are also habitually resolved away by re-establishing the asymmetry (i.e., the divide) between the discursive and material outcomes of participatory development. That is, relativist accounts of participatory development are stated habitually in the face of material outcomes and objective conditions that do not support the account. Instead of tracing action, these accounts (both the universalist and relativist versions) still rely on discursive generalization grounded in rigid foundational distinctions between Science and Society. In the remainder of this book, I endeavor to present a different type of account.

The fundamental asymmetry to be addressed is that participatory development is not routinely observed in practice without re-creating divides and imposing orders that match the discursive ideal of a generalized (or representational) account of participatory development. Mosse (2001), in his critique of participatory development, summarized this asymmetry well:

> [I]t is possible to see that there is an oblique relationship between the rationality of 'participation' policy and the world of practice; to see how projects and programmes shape as well as implement policy; how the language of participation is co-opted from below as much as imposed from above; how there is never a singular voice, or a harmonious consensus around projects; and how power in development is multi-centered, and practices indeterminate and adaptive. A theory of participation separate from analysis of the meaning of the concept in specific organizational practices would be impossible. (Mosse, 2001, 32)

Not all actions are counted as participation. The actions of a great number of people are narrowed to fit the ideal model, even though many diverse actions are necessary for development success and some actions may even be more important than participation, per se. Those projects that most closely express the ideal of participatory development are usually given more attention, and those that do not are routinely overlooked or otherwise explained away. The participation necessary for regular development is made utterly invisible, and the failures of participatory development are held at bay (although some of these failures are now, finally, emerging and being seriously discussed). Thus, a divide between what is endogenous and what is exogenous is constructed, and this leads to an asymmetry between a practice-based understanding and a representational understanding of participatory development.

The dominant way of knowing participation is as a catalyst or cause of better development outcomes; however, the perceived need for participatory development often is the result of previous alienation from development. Consequently, participatory development could be viewed as a symptom of development failure as well as a cause of development success. Multiple definitions of participatory development become possible. Even within a participatory framework where experts descend on a community to facilitate participatory methods, local visions, lay knowledge, and community narratives can be dismissed as unscientific and can be easily ignored. An action-based account of participatory development would reflect increased sensitivity to the quality and outcomes of participation as actually practiced, leading to an ability to differentiate effective participation from business-as-usual wrapped up in a cloak of participatory language and routines that lead to no real change. In other words, rather than representing acts of participation in reference to an idealized image, actions would be traced in detail with an emphasis on describing practice.

To learn from practice we have to drop the grand narratives to which we constantly generalized in the past; the shorthand accounts that freely traveled across space and time to enforce the same label on different actions in different places. Grand narratives could be viewed as tropes rather than as knowledge, per se, not because of their grandness but because they are applied *a priori* to any situation. For example, the notion of *participatory* development pre-assigns an order in which *regular* development exists at the center of reference, and participatory development exists for others located outside that center, begging such questions as "Does people's participation lead to better development outcomes?" In contrast, one could ask "In what situations is participatory development produced?" or "What constitutes participatory development in this event?," thus eliminating the need to separate "regular" development from a development intended for an "other" who is not included and averting the use of participatory development as a trope for producing this divide.

Instead of imagining that participatory development causes people to act collectively, participatory development can be recognized as the effect of the interactions among people and things. This way of thinking is not universalist or relativist; it is a third way, and an attempt to resolve the problems of the first two by questioning how reality gets divided and categorized by asking who are the actors, what is the action, and what is the outcome.[51] An actor/action-oriented approach questions the very source of an explanation and where things are situated. Centers of reference, stances, conventional discourses, units of analysis: these all have to be problematized. The privileged vantage point of a unified conception of participatory development (whether universalist or relativist), contrasted against a highly diverse material reality that is in no way described by a unified conception can no longer be maintained.

Participatory development is an order of thought and practice that has become ubiquitous in the international development realm. On the basis of the premise that conventional development is unable to reach people in the Global South, a participatory development paradigm has emerged as a special way of thinking about and categorizing poor people's development. I challenge the idea that we must necessarily think about poor people's development differently than we think about everyone else's development. Each chapter of this book will demonstrate methods for observing development practice in ways that embrace difference while abolishing asymmetrical accounts on the grounds that they are fundamentally biased.

Organization of the Argument

The overall argument of the book is presented in the remaining six chapters. Chapter 2 introduces and summarizes the wide-reaching reforms that were enacted in Brazil from the 1980s through the 1990s. Brazil's transition to democracy is summarized with special emphasis on the resulting decentralization of government in general, and of the water and sanitation sector in particular. Corresponding with these national and state level reforms was Brazil's sanitation movement, a social movement of grassroots actors in solidarity with professional health care and environmental actors. Chapter 2 also portrays the emergence of a new sanitation technology in the Northeast region of the country. This innovation was introduced by activist engineers as an attempt to extend sanitation service to unserved residents who, because of the influence of the sanitation movement and a new democracy that seemed to welcome their involvement in public decision-making, were organizing around demands for basic infrastructure services. These engineers began to understand not only the technical challenges of expanding sewer service to unserved neighborhoods, but also the social and financial challenges. They developed a new sanitation technology,[52] and through the 1980s and early 1990s they experimented with various ways of implementing the new technology with participation. Chapter 2 fully explains this innovative technology in the context of the multiple levels of reform that were achieved.

With the big picture of reform laid out as a backdrop, chapter 3 introduces the sanitation situation in two cities of Brazil's Northeast region, the first capital cities in the country to experiment with condominial sewerage. The cities of Natal and Recife offer contrasting contexts for observing the birth and proliferation of condominial sewer projects. The urban geography of these two local settings is described, followed by a description of the governance structures that were created to deliver services as well as information about the degree of emergence of condominial sewerage in each city as measured by growth in the number of household connections. The chapter establishes how condominial sewerage began and how much it expanded during the initial innovation period.

In chapter 4, the book tells how multiple actors and actions came together in the city of Natal to produce the first condominial sewer projects, which were variously called simplified, low-cost, condominial, backyard, or sidewalk sewers. The story involves engineers who were willing to champion a new sewer technology and a new participatory approach. These innovations directly challenged the status quo and required the activist engineers to act strategically so they would be allowed the freedom to experiment. The chapter also reveals Natal's response to the decentralizing milieu in which it found itself as the nation was establishing a democracy. Natal is unusual because of its initial resistance to decentralizing its water and sanitation agency and the extent to which the state water and sanitation agency was able to protect the innovation and maintain control over much of the experimentation. The chapter shows how success in this urban setting required the creation and maintenance of an "alignment of interests" to support each individual project.

Chapter 5 describes how condominial sewerage became established in Recife, the second Northeast capital city to adopt the innovation. Although located in the same region as Natal, Recife offers a very different urban setting. The degree of decentralized governance in the sector and the influence of organized communities in Recife led to very different performance outcomes compared to Natal. Recife is a story of battles between competing regimes over how sanitation services should be delivered, what role communities should have in that delivery, and whether or how all communities could be included in the service. The innovation was not controlled by a single entity as in Natal; rather, multiple actors were engaged in the innovation. The chapter explores the complicated relations among multiple actors involved in sanitation development—elected officials, practitioners, residents, and projects—and explains how isolated performance success emerged from these relations. Urban development in Recife was much more complicated and success much more difficult to attain because of the difficulty in forming and maintaining stable project coalitions.

Chapter 6 compares the experiences of Natal and Recife for the purpose of identifying the important themes associated with successful and failed project performance. The key actors are identified in each setting, and the nature of the project coalitions that linked them is analyzed for a selected set of case study projects. The analysis reveals the conditions that led to successful service delivery in each urban setting. Project performance was contingent on the strength and stability of coalitions of elected officials, implementing agencies, and residents. These project coalitions were strong and stable when interests were aligned, when communities had influence, and when residents participated in project-oriented mobilizing and decision-making. The notion of a project coalition aids in understanding why some projects failed and others succeeded, and the comparative case analysis of Natal and Recife reveals the conditions in which project coalitions became either strong and stable or weak and short-lived. The resulting project coalition-based account recognizes the existence of networks that form around infrastructure projects. Project coalitions explain project outcomes more accurately than community participation alone by taking account of the following: 1) different forms of participation impact project outcomes differently; 2) people participate outside the realm of government-designed participation programs; and 3) project outcome is a function not only of program design, but of the conditions of implementation in a specific time and place. While condominial sewer projects were inspired by community participation, in practice it was the strength and stability of project coalitions that were associated with actual project performance.

The concluding chapter, chapter 7, analyzes the development of a discursive paradigm for condominial sewerage, which I call "participatory sanitation." Participatory sanitation as a paradigm is identified through a content analysis of written and oral texts used by the engineers and officials who brought the innovation from Natal and Recife to Bahia, the third Northeast capital city to adopt the condominial sewer innovation. These engineers distilled their varied ideas about and experiences of condominial sewerage into a general conception or paradigm. The paradigm for condominial sewerage did not accurately predict or describe real project experiences, but accuracy in this sense was not necessary for the purpose of enrolling new actors. The chapter points out the overwhelmingly positive orientation and non-critical attitude promoters had toward the participatory sanitation paradigm, and shows how the paradigm was used successfully to persuade other engineers to adopt the technology and to eventually solidify condominial sewerage as a legitimate new technology in Brazil's sanitation sector.

Overview of the Entire Book

During Brazil's transition to democracy (1984–1995), municipalities gained access to federal funding and sought to expand access to public services such as basic sanitation. Corresponding with these reforms in infrastructure funding, the prevailing model for public sanitation service changed from a conventional approach to a participatory approach, which employed lower-cost technology and citizen involvement. This change was significant because it constituted a paradigm shift in service delivery that increased local voice in the sanitation sector. The book describes why and how this new approach varied in different urban contexts, and explores the nature of the coalitions established among elected officials, water and sanitation agencies, communities, and projects in two capital cities in Brazil's Northeast region. Evidence from detailed performance evaluations show that successful outcomes depended largely on project coalitions rather than on people's participation in the projects. These findings challenge the central assumptions of the participatory development paradigm.

Further evidence demonstrates that activist engineers, willing to challenge their own professional discipline and skilled in the discursive use of the participatory sanitation paradigm, successfully transferred the innovation to engineers in other Brazilian cities who adopted the new technology on the basis of this paradigm. But rather than emphasizing formal, rational evaluations of project performance, activist engineers narrated the development outcomes they were trying to promote. In so doing, small, local narratives about actual outcomes in specific places were suppressed and marginalized in favor of a constructed grand narrative that did not describe but rather mythologized the process of condominial sewer development. Their discursive use of the participatory sanitation paradigm was instrumental in attracting new supporters and resources and for developing opportunities to experiment with ways to eventually make the projects work. The utility of narrated development was in extending networks and expanding the space to act. With this essentially political process, activist engineers succeeded in making Brazil's water and sanitation sector more inclusive than it had ever been in the past.

Closing Remarks for Chapter 1

This chapter established that the water and sanitation sector routinely excludes people from service on a global scale, and that Brazil offers a unique and critical case for examining new ways to extend services into unserved and otherwise marginalized neighborhoods. Brazil's innovative approach was consistent with the principles of participation that were adopted by international development organizations, who promoted community participation as a way to improve project performance and serve areas lacking formal infrastructure. However, the asymmetries inherent in community participation make it difficult to construct a useful account of this innovation that does not simply reproduce participation as a trope; consequently, Brazil's experience will be traced using actor-oriented methods. The remainder of the book describes, evaluates, and critiques the rise and spread of this unique innovation in Brazil and explains how and why it was successful.

Notes

1. See, for example, Maria Aycrigg, "Participation and the World Bank: Success, Constraints, and Responses" (Washington, DC: World Bank, 1998).

2. United Nations, "Clean Water and Sanitation for the Poor" 2003, http://www.undp.org/dpa/publications/FSwater120303E.pdf (12 Jan. 2005).

3. The term "majority world" refers to poor and low income people worldwide, while "minority world" refers to the smaller number of wealthier people on the planet (see Nick Lee and Paul Stenner, "Who Pays? Can We Pay Them Back?," in *Actor Network Theory and After*, ed. John Law and John Hassard [Oxford: Blackwell Publishers, 1999]). These terms are not geographically specific and are intended to replace terms such as the Global South and the Global North, thereby recognizing the fact that a great number of marginalized people reside in countries of the Global North. These terms are also intended to overcome the condescension inherent in using terms like Third World.

4. United Nations, *World Urbanization Prospects: The 2001 Revision* 2002, http://www.un.org/esa/population/publications/wup2001/WUP2001report.htm (12 Sep. 2005).

5. World Health Organization, "Global Water Supply and Sanitation Assessment 2000 Report" 2000, http://www.who.int/docstore/water_sanitation_health/Globassess ment/Global1.htm#1.1 (29 Mar. 2004).

6. World Health Organization, "Global Water Supply and Sanitation Assessment 2000 Report" 2000, http://www.who.int/docstore/water_sanitation_health/Globassess ment/Global1.htm#1.1 (29 Mar. 2004); and Steven A. Esrey, James B. Potash, Leslie Roberts, and Clive Shiff, "Quantifying the Health Effects of Water and Sanitation Projects" (Washington, DC: World Bank, 1991).

7. Pan American Health Organization, "Special Program for Health Analysis Linear Interpolation Based on UN Data: World Urbanization Prospects, the 1999 Revision" 1999, www.paho.org (29 Mar. 2004).

8. Instituto Brasileiro de Geografia e Estatística, *Brasil 2001* 2001, www.IBGE.gov.br/english/presidencia/noticias/12062003indic2002.shtm (19 Oct. 2005).

9. Pan American Health Organization, "Country Health Profile–Brazil" in *Health in the Americas* 1998, http://www.paho.org/english/sha/prflbra.htm (29 Mar. 2004).

10. Sandy Cairncross and Richard G. Feachem, *Environmental Health Engineering in the Tropics: An Introductory Text* (Chichester, UK: John Wiley & Sons, 1993) 154.

11. Another promising (and in many ways more sustainable) option is dry composting toilets, which do not require water and could be the most reasonable alternative in situations where water is scarce or intermittent. Urban gardens need to be in place for use of the resulting compost material. See Robert Goodland, Laura Orlando, and Jeff Anhang, *Toward Sustainable Sanitation* 2001, http://riles.org (23 Nov. 2009).

12. Luiz Carlos Rangel Soares, ed., "Regional Report on the Evaluation 2000 in the Region of the Americas: Water Supply and Sanitation, Current Status and Prospects" (Washington, DC: Pan American Health Organization and World Health Organization, 2001), 16–17.

13. Gehan S. Sinnatamby, "Low Cost Sanitation," in *The Poor Die Young: Housing and Health in Third World Cities*, eds. Sandy Cairncross, Jorge E. Hardoy, and David Satterthwaite (London: Earthscan Publications, 1990), 146–47; and Alexander Bakalian and N. Vijay Jagannathan, "Institutional Aspects of the Condominial Sewer System" (Washington, DC: World Bank, 1991).

14. This is not to imply that affluent residents are paying the full costs of the conventional sewer services they receive. On the contrary, conventional systems are typically heavily subsidized by governments, including Brazil's government.

15. A "*salário minimo*" in Brazil is the minimum wage, in *reais* (Brazilian dollars), accumulated over one month. See Instituto Brasileiro de Geografia e Estatística, *Pesquisa Nacional por Amostra de Domicílios* (*National Household Sample Survey*) 2001. http://www.ibge.gov.br/english/presidencia/noticias/12062003indic2002.shtm (29 Mar. 2004), 8.

16. Instituto Brasileiro de Geografia e Estatística, *Brasil 2001* 2001, www.IBGE.gov.br/english/presidencia/noticias/12062003indic2002.shtm (19 Oct. 2005).

17. World Bank, *World Development Report 1994: Infrastructure for Development* (Washington, DC: Oxford University Press, 1994), 22–25.

18. Miguel Vargas-Ramirez and Teresa Cristina Lampoglia, "Scaling-up Using Condominial Technology," *Waterlines* 25, no. 2 (2006): 12.

19. José M. Azevedo-Netto, "Innovative and Low Cost Technologies Utilized in Sewerage" (Washington, DC: Pan American Health Organization and World Health Organization, 1992), 48; and World Bank, *World Development Report 1992: Development and the Environment* (Washington, DC: Oxford University Press, 1992), 107. Also, Bakalian, et al. reported average capital costs of conventional sewers in Brazil (in 1988 U.S. dollars) ranging from US$150 to $300 per capita, not including house connections, wastewater treatment, system maintenance, and disposal costs (see Alexander Bakalian, Albert Wright, Richard Otis, and José M. Azevedo-Netto, *Simplified Sewerage: Design Guidelines* (Washington, DC: The World Bank, 1994), 19.

20. Sheldon Annis and Peter Hakim, eds., *Direct to the Poor: Grassroots Development in Latin America* (Boulder and London: Lynne Rienner Publishers, 1988).

21. Gehan Sinnatamby, "Low Cost Sanitation Systems for Urban Peripheral Areas in Northeast Brazil," Ph.D. dissertation (Leeds, UK: The University of Leeds, 1983).

22. John Briscoe and Harvey A. Garn, "Financing Water Supply and Sanitation Under Agenda 21" *Natural Resources Forum* 19, no. 1 (1995): 59–70.

23. Briscoe and Garn, *Natural Resources Forum*, 59–70.

24. Mary Elmendorf and Patricia Buckles, "Sociocultural Aspects of Water Supply and Excreta Disposal," *Appropriate Technology for Water Supply and Sanitation* 5 (Washington, DC: The World Bank, 1980).

25. Richard A. Gorell, "Families in Shantytowns in Sao Paulo, Brazil, 1945–1984: The Rural-Urban Connection," Ph.D. dissertation (Lawrence, KS: University of Kansas, 1990).

26. See, for example, Jonathan Isham, Deepa Narayan, and Lant Pritchett, "Does Participation Improve Performance? Establishing Causality with Subjective Data," *World Bank Economic Review* 9, no. 2 (1995): 175–200; Deepa Narayan, "The Contribution of People's Participation: Evidence from 121 Rural Water Supply Projects" (Washington, DC: The World Bank, 1995); Gabrielle Watson and N. Vijay Jagannathan, "Participation in Water and Sanitation" (Washington, DC: The World Bank, 1995); Elinor Ostrom, "Crossing the Great Divide: Co-Production, Synergy, and Development, "*World Development* 24, no. 6 (1996): 1073–88; Albert Wright, "Toward a Strategic Sanitation Approach: Improving the Sustainability of Urban Sanitation in Developing Countries" (Washington, DC: The World Bank, 1997); Linda S. Prokopy, "The Relationship between Participation and Project Outcomes: A Study of Rural Drinking Water Projects in India," Ph.D. dissertation (Chapel Hill, NC: University of North Carolina, 2002); and World Bank, *World Development Report 2004: Making Services Work for Poor People* (Washington, DC: Oxford University Press, 2004).

27. Earthea Nance, "Putting Participation in Context: An Evaluation of Urban Sanitation in Brazil," Ph.D. dissertation (Stanford, CA: Stanford University, 2004); and Earthea Nance and Leonard Ortolano, "Community Participation in Urban Sanitation: Experiences in Northeastern Brazil," *Journal of Planning Education and Research* 26 (2007): 284–300.

28. Household interviews were conducted with the help of local research assistants.

29. Lant Pritchett and Michael Woolcock, "Solutions when *the* Solution Is the Problem: Arraying the Disarray in Development," *World Development* 32, no. 2 (2004): 206–7.

30. See, for example, Bruno Latour, *We Have Never Been Modern* (Cambridge, MA: Harvard University Press, 1993); Helen Verran, *Science and an African Logic* (Chicago and London: The University of Chicago Press, 2001); and Annemarie Mol, 'Ontological Politics: A Word and Some Questions," in *Actor Network Theory and After*, eds., John Law and John Hassard (Oxford: Blackwell Publishers, 1999).

31. Development with a capital "D" refers to dominant discourses of development as expressed, for example, by James Ferguson, *The Anti-Politics Machine: "Development," Depoliticization, and Bureaucratic Power in Lesotho* (New York: Cambridge University Press, 1990); Wolfgang Sachs, ed., *The Development Dictionary: A Guide to Knowledge as Power* (London and New York: Zed Books, 1992); and Arturo Escobar, *Encountering Development: The Making and Unmaking of the Third World* (Princeton, NJ: Princeton University Press, 1995).

32. Mark Hobart, ed., *Discourses of Development: Anthropological Perspectives* (London and New York: Routledge, 1993), 1.

33. See, for example, R. D. Grillo, "Discourses of Development: The View from Anthropology," in *Discourses of Development: Anthropological Perspectives*, eds. R. D. Grillo and R. L. Stirrat (Oxford: Berg, 1997), 19–27.

34. See, for example, Grillo, "Discourses of Development," 24–25.

35. See, for example, Stephen Healy, "Toward a Vocabulary for Speaking of the Engagement of Things into Discourse," *Journal of Environmental Policy and Planning* 7, no. 3 (2005): 248; and David Mosse, "People's Knowledge, Participation, and Patronage: Operations and Representations in Rural Development," in *Participation: The New Tyranny?*, eds. Bill Cooke and Uma Kothari (London and New York: Zed Books, 2001), 31.

36. Cooke and Kothari, *Participation: The New Tyranny?*; and Ricardo Toledo Silva, "Urban Reconstruction and Institutional Reshaping in Brazil," in *The Challenge of Sustainable Cities: Neoliberalism and Urban Strategies in Developing Countries*, eds. Rod Burgess, Marisa Carmona, and Theo Kolstee (London and New Jersey: Zed Books, 1997), 181.

37. World Bank, "Latin American and Caribbean Seminar on Water and Sanitation for Low-Income Groups" (Washington, DC: World Bank, 1989) and World Bank, *World Development Report 2004*.

38. Janice Perlman, *The Myth of Marginality: Urban Politics and Poverty in Rio de Janeiro* (Berkeley, CA: University of California Press, 1976), 121.

39. Alfredo Luiz Buso, Katia Mello, and Marcos Costa Lima, "Integrated Urban Development: The Dike Project in Santos," in *The Challenge of Sustainable Cities: Neoliberalism and Urban Strategies in Developing Countries*, eds. Rod Burgess, Marisa Carmona, and Theo Kolstee (London and New Jersey: Zed Books, 1997), 209.

40. Pritchett and Woolcock, "Solutions when *the* Solution Is the Problem," 197.

41. Birgitte Hoffmann, Susanne Balslev Nielsen, Morton Elle, Soren Gabriel, Anne Marie Eilersen, Mogens Henze, and Peter Steen Mikellsen, "Assessing the Sustainability of Small Wastewater Systems: A Context-Oriented Planning Approach," *Environmental Impact Assessment Review* 20 (2000): 350.

42. Sachs, *The Development Dictionary*; Ferguson, *The Anti-Politics Machine*; Escobar, *Encountering Development*; Arturo Escobar, "Planning," in *The Development Dictionary: A Guide to Knowledge as Power*, ed. Wolfgang Sachs (London and New York: Zed Books, 1992); and Trevor Parfitt, *The End of Development* (London: Pluto Press, 2002).

43. The terms "minority world" and "majority world" are borrowed from Lee and Stenner, "Who Pays? Can We Pay Them Back?," 105.

44. Cooke and Kothari, *Participation: The New Tyranny?*.

45. Sherry R. Arnstein, "A Ladder of Citizen Participation," *Journal of the American Institute of Planners* 35, no. 4 (1969): 216–24.

46. Marisa B. Guaraldo Choguill, "A Ladder of Community Participation for Underdeveloped Countries," *Habitat International* 20, no. 3 (1996): 431–44.

47. Diane Day, "Citizen Participation in the Planning Process: An Essentially Contested Concept?," *Journal of Planning Literature* 11, no. 3 (1997): 421–34.

48. See, for example, Verran, *Science and an African Logic*.

49. Latour, *We Have Never Been Modern*.

50. See, for example, Latour, *We Have Never Been Modern*; Lee and Stenner "Who Pays? Can We Pay Them Back?," 95; Mol, "Ontological Politics;" and Annemarie Mol, *The Body Multiple: Multiple Realities in Medicine*, 2003.

51. Bruno Latour, "The Powers of Association," in *Power, Action, and Belief: A New Sociology of Knowledge?*, ed. John Law (London: Routledge & Kegan Paul, 1986), 264–80; Bruno Latour, *Politics of Nature: How to Bring the Sciences into Democracy* (Cambridge, MA: Harvard University Press, 2004); Verran, *Science and an African Logic*; Healey, "Toward a Vocabulary for Speaking of the Engagement of Things into Discourse"; and Grillo, "Discourses of Development."

52. In Brazil, this technology is called *sistema de esgoto condominial*, which literally translates to "condominial sewer system" in English. A more meaningful translation of this phrase is a collective or community-based sewer system in which an organized group of residents participates in delivering the service. Condominial sewer systems are based on the principles of participatory development—or, to be more specific, "participatory sanitation."

Chapter 2
Institutional Change, Social Movements, and Technological Innovation in Brazil

Institutional changes are necessary if the promise of participatory development is to be realized. This chapter introduces and summarizes the wide-reaching reforms that were enacted in Brazil from the 1980s through the 1990s. Brazil's transition to democracy is summarized with special emphasis on the resulting decentralization of government in general and of the water and sanitation sector in particular. Corresponding with these national and state level reforms was Brazil's sanitation movement, a social movement of grassroots groups in solidarity with health care and environmental professionals. The chapter also notes the emergence of a new sanitation technology in the Northeast region of the country as an attempt by activist engineers to address the technical, social, and financial challenges of expanding sewer service. These engineers developed a more appropriate sanitation technology, and through the 1980s and early 1990s they experimented with various ways of implementing the new technology. The chapter describes this innovative technology in the context of the multiple levels of reform that were in process.

Democratizing and Decentralizing Brazil

One of the first and most important steps toward democracy in Brazil was the establishment of electoral voting. Prior to democratization, state governors had been appointed by the president of Brazil. But beginning in 1982 state governors were directly elected by popular vote, and in 1985 the popular election of city mayors was established. These changes allowed more reform politicians to attain executive positions where they could initiate policies and programs to improve and expand urban services. For example, in the state of Pernambuco, populist opposition candidate Miguel Arraes won the 1987 gubernatorial election and subsequently enacted policies and programs to serve his political base, which largely consisted of poor and working class people. Prior to these popular elections, most government agencies involved in service provision did not have the political space to proactively expand urban services on their own. Service provision had been largely clientelistic and exploitive, or merely a reaction to large mobilizations of citizens and immediate political pressure.[1] As the democratic transition continued and as populist politicians were elected, governmental implementing organizations (e.g., water and sanitation companies, housing agencies, urban planning departments, etc.) were more able to initiate periods of planned expansion of urban services. These periods of proactive implementation were often preceded by the election of a populist executive-level politician who supported the proposals of progressive technical employees within the implementing organizations. The democratic transition also brought the potential for wide swings in political administrations with each election cycle that, in some locations, resulted in discontinuous support for urban service projects from one administration to the next. But the biggest impact on the water and sanitation sector was decentralization.

Brazil had centralized its water and sanitation sector in the early 1970s under President Medici's administration. The country had adopted a state enterprise institutional model, whereby the federal government created and directly funded large state-owned companies that specialized in the implementation of water and sanitation infrastructure in each state. Under these institutional arrangements, project decision-making had been centralized at the state level. Most water and sanitation investments of the 1970s and 1980s had been channeled to the state water and sanitation companies through Brazil's National Sanitation Plan (*Plano Nacional de Saneamento*, or PLANASA), which had been funded by the National Housing Bank (*Banco Nacional da Habita□ão*, or BNH).[2] From 1970 to 1989, PLANASA provided R$11.3 billion in federal funding to state water and sanitation companies for infrastructure projects throughout Brazil.[3] The majority of PLANASA-era funds supported water development, because at that time the need for water projects was perceived to be higher than the need for sanitation projects. Funds from international donors and lending agencies (such as the World Bank) also had been channeled through the BNH for distribution to state water and sanitation companies and to municipalities that implemented the projects.[4]

Table 2-1 presents estimates of the percentage of the Brazilian population with access to water and sewer service from 1970 to 2011. The estimates in Table 2-1 illustrate the great increases in water and sewer access achieved during the PLANASA-era peak (1970-1989); and access rates at the end of the PLANASA era (1991), discounting the erroneous estimates of 1995. Table 2-1 also shows that investments in conventional sewers consistently lagged behind investments in water supply. However, most of these impressive investments did not reach the poor. Silva et al. (1996) concluded that Brazil's sanitation development policy was limited to "formal, legitimate urban areas,"[5] which effectively excluded poor people by definition.[6] Parlatore characterizes the outcome of the PLANASA era as follows:[7]

> Despite PLANASA's major achievements, the institution failed to accomplish universal service, especially in the poorest regions . . . in the North and Northeast. . . . Rural-urban migration grew considerably during the period in which PLANASA was in effect, causing rapid and disorderly growth at the outskirts of medium and large cities and making it increasingly difficult and expensive to provide water supply and sewerage services in such areas.

Table 2-1. Estimated access to piped water supply and sanitary sewer services in Brazil from 1970 to 2011. (See footnote regarding 1995 data.)

Year	Access to Piped Water (% of population)	Access to Sewers (% of population)
1970	55–60%	22%
1980	72%	21% [a]
1991	86%	49%
1995	91% [b]	66% [b]
1999	83.9%	41.2%
2005	82.3%	69.7%
2011	84.6%	62.6%

Sources: Parlatore, undated; IBGE, 1999; IBGE PNAD, 1999, 2005, and 2011; World Bank, 1994; and Cardoso, 1989, 305.

a. The figures for 1980 are sewer or septic tank access from the World Bank (1994) and Cardoso (1989:305). Figures for the remaining years are for sewer access only.

b. The inconsistent pattern of improvement in water and sewer access between 1995 and 1999 indicates the possibility of a high level of error in establishing how much of the population was being served at any given time. PAHO/WHO (2001, 44) reported that Brazil's 1995 water and sewer access estimates were likely too high due to errors in population estimates.

The institutional arrangements that had been set up in the 1970s included federal rules that declared municipal governments had control over local water and sanitation development. The great majority of Brazilian cities had subcontracted their water and sanitation development in twenty-year contracts with the new state-owned water and sanitation companies. These contracts assigned to state water companies the job of providing infrastructure services to cities, but some cities were more dependent on the water companies than others. Because the water and sanitation companies were state-owned, they were often politically tied to the governor of their respective state who appointed their director. The water and sanitation companies were impacted by political differences between the state governor (to whom they were directly tied) and the capital city mayor (with whom they often had their largest contracts). Small, rural interior towns and medium-sized cities tended to be in a position of deep dependence on the state. Large, wealthy capital cities, however, had some capacity to act independently, as demonstrated by periods in which they contended with the state over water and sanitation policy and program implementation. As state governors moved funds away from the urban centers and toward the more needy interior, capital cities either enhanced their relationship with the state or made attempts to develop their own water and sanitation sector and provide services independently (these dynamics are further elaborated in chapter 4).

As part of Brazil's democratic transition, the new Constitution of 1988 changed public infrastructure financing from the highly centralized PLANASA-style system to a largely decentralized scheme.[8] Under the new decentralized financing scheme, federal money for local infrastructure services (including World Bank loans, etc.) would be distributed directly to municipalities rather than through the state water and sanitation companies. This new arrangement would, effectively, alter the balance of power between cities and states. Municipalities would be able to either build and manage their own water and sanitation projects, hire private companies, or hire the state water and sanitation company to implement, operate, and maintain city water and sewer services. An engineer in one city's municipal urbanization agency described the impact of these changes as follows:[9]

> During the dictatorship, everything was concentrated and centralized, and CAERN [the state water and sanitation agency] did everything. Then this all changed and things became decentralized in 1988. Part of this process included deciding what responsibilities would be transferred to the municipalities and what CAERN would continue doing. . . . The problem is that the City wants CAERN to do more and CAERN wants the City to do more. Another problem is that all of the technical staff and expertise is in CAERN.

The new decentralized finance arrangements were put into practice by President Itamar in the early 1990s. Since that time, cities have been able to acquire their own funds and implement sanitation projects (including condominial sewer projects) without necessarily involving the state water and sanitation companies, and the water companies have had to obtain agreements with city governments before they could receive project money. In essence, decentralization triggered state water companies to begin marketing their services to city governments, sometimes in competition with private companies. The evolving balance of power between capital cities and the state (via decentralization) and between elected officials and citizens (via democratization) had important implications for the implementation of water and sanitation services and on the capacity and willingness of engineers and their implementing organizations to expand services to poor residents.

Brazil's Sanitation Movement

Part of Brazil's democratic transition included what Gerschman (1993) called a "sanitation movement." This movement consisted of grassroots popular movements of poor residents and middle-class movements of health workers and doctors who protested, demonstrated, mobilized, lobbied, and otherwise struggled for better public health policies, programs, and facilities.[10] The term "grassroots popular movements," a subset of urban social movements, refers to mobilization of the popular classes (i.e., the poor and the working class).[11] Public health problems, rapid urbanization, the growing lack of urban services such as water and sanitation, and the political opening (i.e., democratization) of the late 1970s and early 1980s motivated numerous popular and middle-class movements to focus on environmental health issues. The influence of these movements, identified collectively as the sanitation movement, corresponded with new attitudes about the urbanization and integration of poor neighborhoods and shantytowns (known as *favelas* in Brazil) into cities as opposed to the previous policy of demolition.[12] The sanitation movement also set the stage for the emergence of new attitudes about conventional sewer technology. Before the sanitation movement, conventional sewer technology from highly industrialized countries had been accepted as the primary sewerage solution. After the sanitation movement, sewer officials and engineers throughout Brazil began to question the appropriateness of conventional sewer technology[13] and showed a new willingness to experiment with condominial sewer technology. This willingness and the subsequent emergence of condominial sewerage was borne of the struggles of the sanitation movement and the growth of organized neighborhoods.

Table 2-2. Tactics used by Brazilian community-based organizations to mobilize and express demands.

Grassroots Tactics for Expressing Demand in Brazil
Mobilizing large numbers of residents
Conducting sit-ins
Protesting at the doorsteps of government agencies
Signing petitions
Submitting complaints
Inviting government representatives to tour their neighborhoods to witness living conditions
Using the threat of mass protest to force negotiation
Negotiating with officials in small groups
Prioritizing needs and focusing on each one in sequence
Targeting specific demands to appropriate agencies

Source: Watson, 1992.

Rather than organizing around class, Brazilian residents tended to organize around residential location (i.e., neighborhoods).[14] Residents formed community-based organizations (CBOs) that demanded water, sewer, housing, pavement, electricity, and other urban services from elected officials and government agencies. They used a variety of tactics in their struggles for service (see Table 2-2).[15]

Although grassroots mobilizing alone did not reform local and state implementing organizations, it did play at least three important roles. Mobilizing allowed residents to express their basic needs to reformist officials, to exert pressure on implementing organizations, and to trigger collaboration between residents and implementing organizations in seeking viable service solutions.[16] Even more important than the mobilizing tactics used by different community-based organizations was the political rationale behind their organizing activity.

Prior to the democratic transition, community-based organizations in poor neighborhoods were integrated into local-level clientelistic politics, in which large populations of poor residents that were organized at the neighborhood level served as inexpensive sources of votes for politicians.[17] The clientele system was deeply entrenched throughout Brazil. Even though clientelism exploited the poor and perpetuated their dependent and powerless situation, it provided short-term advantages for both the patron and the client.[18] The client/community would receive desperately needed services—usually right around election time—and their patron/politician would gain a block of votes. Larger neighborhoods had more potential votes and thus had more influence, so they were in a better position to bargain for better services. Watson (1992) argued that in Sao Paulo collaboration between residents and implementing organizations was an effective strategy and was not merely an act of cooptation by the state.[19] Mainwaring (1989) also elaborated on the complexity of this relationship as follows:[20]

> Although it is important for social movements to avoid becoming a servile instrument of parties or politicians, it is also important that they influence political parties and the State. What is sometimes portrayed as cooptation may be good judgment on the part of movement leaders. . . . A discussion of autonomy/cooptation should therefore focus on trade-offs rather than simply positing the importance of "autonomy" in some undefined sense.

Community organizing was necessary so that the president of a community association could assess the most pressing needs of the residents and announce which politician was to receive everyone's vote. Clientele-oriented organizing activities functioned to reduce transaction costs for the patron, and transferred most of the benefits of empowerment to the community president, whose local prestige and power depended on his or her deal-making ability. The community benefited from this arrangement by receiving neighborhood improvements. However, most of these improvements were one-time gifts rather than long-term services.[21]

Clientelism tended to flourish in local-level politics (rather than in state-level politics). It was not until the democratic transition that the possibility for new forms of community organizing and party politics emerged at the local level.[22] Rather than voting for candidates based on an optimal short-term transaction, democracy-oriented neighborhoods organized to vote for the political party that would represent their needs more broadly. As documented by Gay (1990) in Rio de Janeiro, this new rationale for grassroots organizing in the 1980s was successful in bringing long-term urban services to poor areas in a much more emancipatory and less-exploitive fashion. In the following statement, Gay distinguishes populism from clientelism:[23]

> Populism represents an appeal by political elites to popular discontent with the distribution of power in society. In a sense, populism is simply a more sophisticated form of clientelism in that both represent strategies for the political incorporation of the masses. But although populism is essentially an exchange of "votes for patronage" in that the distribution of benefits is calculated on the basis of what is necessary for consolidating political power, populism is less transactional and more ideological than clientelism.

Mainwaring (1989, 1986) and others have noted that Brazil's democratic opening resulted in increased clientelism and populism.[24] In theory, a democratic system allows poor residents to participate in the political process without being exploited; but democracy in practice can be aimed at pacifying and demobilizing grassroots popular movements rather than empowering them. A clientele system promises to bring immediate benefits to the community, to the community president, and to the politician; hence, the temptation to fall back on clientelism is strong for everyone involved, and the system is difficult to change with or without democracy.

Despite the practical success of Brazil's sanitation movement, some social movement theorists have argued that grassroots popular movements were not likely to have a lasting impact in Brazil. Boschi (1984) found that participation in mobilizing activities increased the participation of residents in the electoral process; that the grassroots movements brought pressure for more democratic and pluralistic social interactions; and that these new social patterns weakened the long-standing clientele system.[25] However, the legitimacy of grassroots organizations as political actors and the institutionalization of permanent channels of access did not occur for at least two reasons. Community organizing was often based on specific, transitory demands; and grassroots popular movements tended to become captured by the government. Community mobilizing that revolves around specific services is considered a transitory demand. Once the service is provided, the demand goes away and the incentive to mobilize disappears. Grassroots organizations that centered their mobilizing activities on attracting new urban services, while sometimes effective in a practical sense, were limited in their ability to make more permanent changes as a social movement. The capture, or cooptation, of individual grassroots organizations by government therefore limited the overall strength of the sanitation movement.

The sanitation movement did succeed in at least one important way. In focusing attention on the environmental health of poor people, the sanitation movement was successful in encouraging new attitudes (e.g., among politicians, government officials, planners, and engineers) about land tenure and service standards that would make it possible to expand urban services to poor neighborhoods. But social movements and new attitudes alone did not trigger the emergence of condominial sewers. Brazil's carefully staged transition to democratic popular elections and decentralized governance would also influence the ways in which urban water and sanitation services were provided.

The Emergence of Condominial Sewerage

In the early 1980s, a new approach to implementing urban services emerged for reaching and including the poor.[26] Case studies of water and sanitation projects had led to a growing policy consensus that approaches involving participation increased the opportunity for service provision to the poor.[27] David Korten and others contended at the time that low-income areas benefited more from "participation approaches" that were characterized by low-technology infrastructure conceived from the perspective of the community itself.[28] Decades of development experience suggested that lower costs, relaxed technical standards, participation, and a localized institutional approach were fundamental aspects of implementing successful projects in low-income areas.[29] The new participatory approaches generally involved some combination of simple, low-cost equipment and local materials; lower design and construction standards; labor-intensive rather than equipment-intensive installation and maintenance techniques; a localized or decentralized approach that could fine-tune projects to each local situation; affordable user fees; and participation of users in identifying local needs, formulating solutions, and implementing projects. An entire line of literature on these approaches (known as "participatory," "bottom-up," "community-based," or "grassroots" development) and technologies (called "appropriate" or "intermediate" technologies) emerged. Brazil's new approach to sanitation—called *condominial* sewers—adopted these principles.

Before the development of condominial sewers in Brazil, relaxed sewer design and construction standards had been practiced widely under the concept of "simplified" sewerage, and the idea of installing collective sewers in yards, alleys, and pathways had been previously tried in India.[30] The use of participation also had been previously established as a beneficial aspect of rural water development in many developing countries. Condominial sewerage brought these two practices—simplified design and participation—together. José Carlos Rodrigues de Melo, a Brazilian civil engineer, is credited with introducing condominial sewers to Brazil and for successfully encouraging and promoting the technology. He estimates that his projects have served millions of people.[31] Melo is also the primary inventor of the condominial sewer paradigm. Among sanitation professionals in Brazil, Melo is known as the "father" of the condominial sewer approach. However, several other Brazilian civil engineers were also at the forefront of developing, promoting, and implementing condominial se wers and creating and disseminating the condominial sewer model. Most notable among these were the academics José M. de Azevedo Netto and Cicero Onofre de Andrade Neto, and the public officials Josemar Azevedo and Maria Geny Formiga de Farias.

Much of the initial innovation and research about condominial sewers was conducted in the State of Rio Grande do Norte by the state water and sanitation agency (*Companhia de Águas e Esgotos do Rio Grande do Norte*, or CAERN) in consultation with professors from the Federal University of Rio Grande do Norte (*Universidade Federal do Rio Grande do Norte*, or UFRN) and the World Bank.[32] In 1978, the state water and sanitation agency (CAERN) had planned to construct a pump station and conventional sewer system in the poor neighborhoods of Rocas and Santos Reis, Natal. But the residents did not have the resources to connect to the proposed system and very few expressed any interest in connecting. Moreover, only six hundred of the homes could be served if the available funding had been used for conventional sewers. To resolve this problem, Melo was called to Natal as a consultant. He proposed a pilot project to determine if a simplified sewer could serve all three thousand homes with the same funds. At that time simplified backyard sewers, sidewalk sewers, and solids-free sewers[33] were only known to exist outside of Brazil.[34]

In 1980, CAERN applied for and received World Bank funds from BNH/PLANASA to implement a pilot project—Brazil's first condominial sewer—in the neighborhoods of Rocas and Santos Reis, Natal. The president of CAERN (Josemar Azevedo) assembled a handful of interested civil and environmental engineers and formed a specialized condominial sewer group to lead the pilot project. Community participation was not an important factor in the initial pilot project and residents did not (and were not expected to) participate in project planning, design, or construction. Technology considerations such as relaxed design standards and affordable materials were the primary concern. The agency did implement a participation program to educate and orient the beneficiaries to their new sewer system; however, this was a far more limited version of participation than would emerge later. CAERN built the street sewer, the condominial sewer, and the house connections. Reflecting on their first project, CAERN engineering staff reported that the Rocas and Santos Reis systems were initially "well-designed" and that the engineers were "very detailed and careful." To emphasize the high standard of care, staff mentioned that the engineers used a survey instrument to confirm the field elevations and to design the location of the condominial sewers and cleanout boxes.[35]

Nevertheless, during the construction of the pilot project the layout of the sewer had to be completely changed. The careful work the engineers had done during design was futile for those parts of the condominial sewer that were located on private property; these sections of the system had to be re-designed in ways that were agreeable to the property owners. From this experience, CAERN learned that the final layout of the condominial sewer and the final location of the cleanout boxes on private property had to be made in the field with the consultation of residents. Design and construction activities could not be separated into two distinct phases; rather, they had to be combined and residents had to be involved.[36] The traditional concept of the project cycle whereby design was distinct from construction and engineers made all of the decisions did not work well in the context of condominial sewers because of their location on private property.

The results of CAERN's initial pilot project in Natal and of its first full-scale condominial sewer projects in several interior towns of the state of Rio Grande do Norte (e.g., in Currais Novos, Parelhas, and Goianinha) were published in a doctoral dissertation,[37] in several volumes of research reports by CAERN, in engineering conference proceedings, and in professional civil and environmental engineering journals. These initial reports helped engineers develop simple design standards for condominial sewers, and established participation as a key part of the condominial sewer implementation approach. Through these experiences, participation became increasingly important to the project. Many beneficiaries were unfamiliar with the proper use and operation of the systems or even the benefits of sewerage.[38] Participation provided a means to introduce the technology and educate the users.

Although condominial sewerage had now emerged, its conception was not yet solidified and the discourse that would sustain it was still in its early stages. The name of the approach was not yet settled. The technology was variously known as simplified sewers, shallow sewers, small bore sewers, condominial sewers, tertiary sewerage, low cost sanitation systems, and backyard sewers,[39] The notion of participation had not yet been firmly linked to the technology, and the technology itself was largely considered experimental.[40] In these early stages (early and mid-1980s), two primary features made condominial sewers stand apart from conventional sewers: relaxed sewer design standards (and the lower costs that resulted) and the installation of the system on private or semi-private property (in lanes, backyards, and front yards). These features were emphasized because they allowed engineers to contrast condominial sewers with what they already knew (i.e., conventional sewers), and because design and siting constraints fit squarely within engineers' existing epistemological framework for thinking about sewers. Eventually, various ideas about condominial sewers came to be represented as a unified concept removed from any context. In the following representational account of condominial sewers, the original emphasis on simple design standards and flexible siting remains. Although it is my own account, other similar accounts are available for this time period.[41]

Layout

Figure 2-1 compares typical piping layouts for condominial and conventional sewers in a planned housing settlement (i.e., a city block). Under a conventional sewer piping layout, sewage from each house is discharged individually to a public sewer in the street. But under "backyard" and "front yard" condominial sewer layouts, a common pipe collects sewage from each group of homes or each city block, which then discharges to a public sewer in the street or other disposal destination (e.g., local septic tank, storm drain, or water body). In the "sidewalk" condominial sewer layout the collection pipe is on public

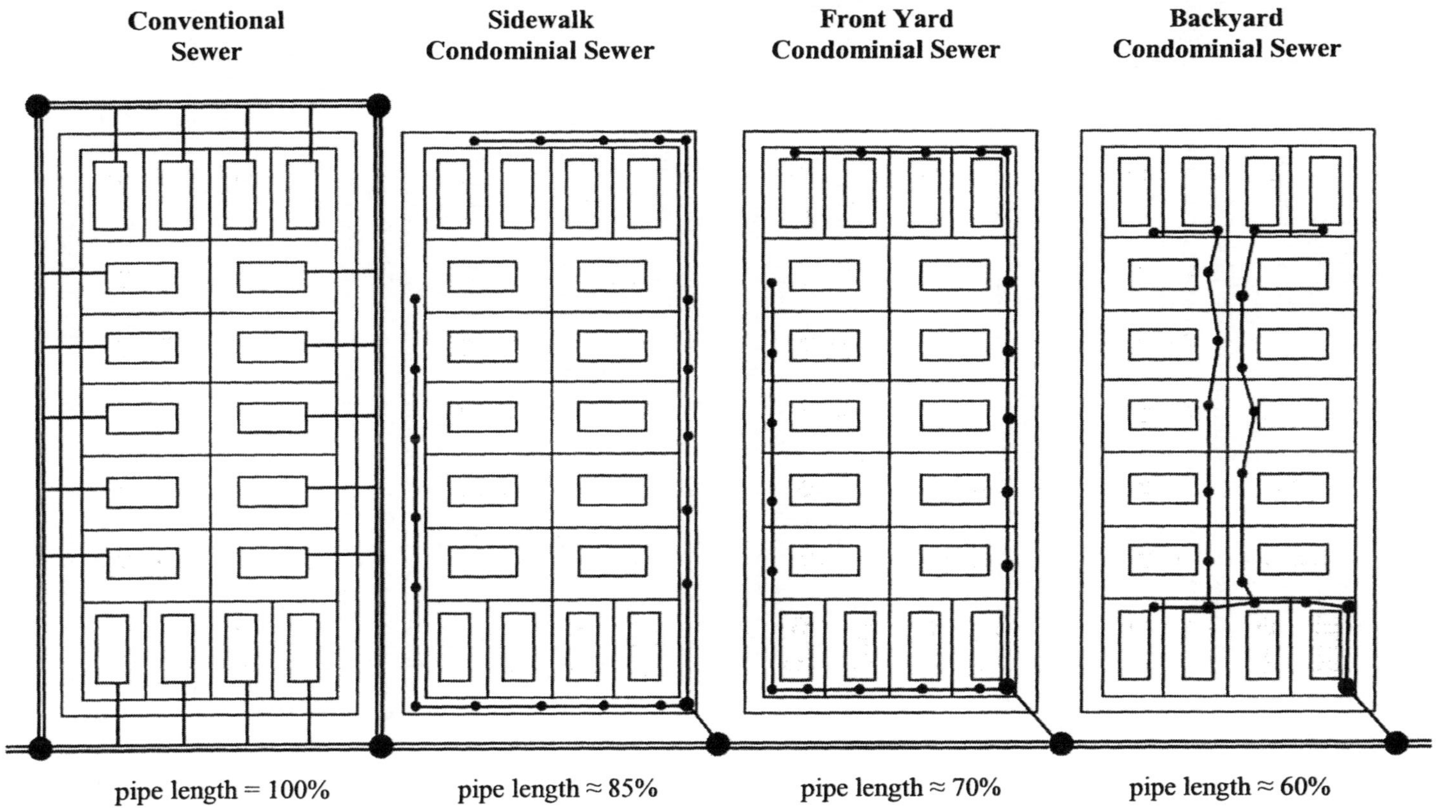

Figure 2-1. Typical piping layouts for conventional and condominial sewer systems.

property—in the sidewalk—and houses discharge their wastewater individually to the sidewalk sewer. The typical boundary between the public and private parts of a condominial sewer system is the most downstream cleanout box, through which all of the wastewater collected from the block flows. Prior to this point, the system is on private property (except in the sidewalk layout). Downstream from this point the system is on public property.

Condominial sewerage requires significantly less pipe (approximately 15 to 40 percent less) than conventional sewerage, which lowers installation costs (see Figure 2-1). When the common collection pipe is installed in the backyards of homes, the overall length of sewer pipe is minimized, resulting in the lowest cost layout. When the common collection pipe is installed in the front yard or sidewalk area of homes, overall pipe length and installation costs are somewhat higher compared to the backyard layout, but costs are still significantly lower than the piping requirements of conventional sewerage.

Cost

Costs vary widely depending on the discharge location, on whether sewage pumping and treatment is included, and on the effect of inflation at the time of the project.[42] In 1993, the World Bank reported capital costs for condominial sewers ranging from US$48 to US$123 per capita for projects in several Brazilian cities (roughly equivalent to $76 to $196 per capita in 2012 US dollars).[43] Overall, the installation cost of condominial sewers ranges from 50 to 80 percent of the installation cost of conventional sewers.[44] During the 1980-2005 time period, capital costs were often spread out over several years to make condominial sewer systems affordable to more residents. The monthly fee charged to Brazilian households for ongoing maintenance of a conventional sewer was typically 100 percent of the household water bill. Typical monthly fees for condominial sewers in Recife and Natal were 80 percent of the water bill for the sidewalk layout, and 40 percent of the water bill for the backyard or front yard layout. The rationale behind this fee structure was that more of the sewer system was located on private property under the backyard and front yard layouts; therefore, project beneficiaries were responsible for maintaining these parts of the sewer system. Because the private parts of the condominial sewer typically did not receive maintenance service by the public sewer authority, lower fees were charged to beneficiaries of backyard and front yard systems. Beneficiaries of sidewalk condominial sewers were charged higher fees because more of their system was located on public property. However, because the sidewalk sewer was not as costly as a conventional sewer, its fee was somewhat lower. The rationale for this fee structure was not based on true maintenance costs. Setting maintenance fees as a percentage of the water bill provided an incentive for residents to connect to sewer service. But this fee system ignored the fact that sewer systems were often more costly to maintain than water systems.[45]

Design

Conventional engineering standards and design criteria are relaxed (or simplified) for condominial sewers. For this reason, condominial sewers are also called "simplified" sewers, "shallow" sewers, or "low-cost" sewers. Condominial sewers are characterized by inexpensive pipe materials, shallow excavations, small diameter pipes, modest slopes, and by their applicability to either planned or unplanned housing settlements. Because condominial sewers can be located in yards, sidewalks, pathways, lanes, or alleys instead of streets, the sewer pipes are not expected to support vehicle loads. Therefore, they can be installed in shallower excavations with lower cost materials. Moreover, smaller overall lengths of pipe are needed to serve a given number of homes with a condominial sewer, as shown previously. Condominial sewer pipe diameters are smaller than typical conventional designs. The standard diameter of a condominial sewer pipe is 100 millimeters (mm), although 150 mm diameter is also used in some locations. The standard diameter of conventional sewer pipe is 150 to 200 mm. These relaxed design standards yield significant cost savings.

Table 2-3 shows a comparison of typical design criteria for condominial sewers and conventional sewers. Sinnatamby (1990) cites sewer field studies that found no association between flatter slopes and the frequency of blockages, and he concluded that "shallow sewer design seeks to maximize the frequency of [sewage] discharges to increase the efficiency with which solids are transported in small diameter pipes."[46]

In a technical review of design criteria for condominial sewers (which the authors also call simplified sewers and shallow sewers), Bakalian et al. concluded that the use of flatter slopes and the relaxation of other sewer design standards to achieve cost savings did not necessarily mean a substandard design. Rather, Bakalian et al. reported that condominial sewers represented a rational alternative "based on sound engineering principles without sacrificing quality or lowering the level of service."[47] In other words, there was no technical reason to believe that condominial sewers should perform poorly just because they were based on relaxed design standards. Nevertheless, Bakalian et al. (1994) did acknowledge that sewer professionals expected simplified sewers to have lower levels of performance and increased maintenance requirements (probably as a result of poor workmanship and misuse).[48]

Installation

The installation of condominial sewers is considerably different from conventional sewer installation. Conventional sewers are typically installed in advance of homes and streets, and individual connections to the conventional sewer are usually installed later as homes are built. The government or the developer can build trunk sewers without any involvement of the residents, and when the

Table 2-3. Typical design criteria for condominial sewers compared to those of conventional sewers[a, d].

Design Item	Typical Condominial Sewer Design Standards	Typical Conventional Sewer Design Standards
Design Period	15–20 years	25–50 years
Peaking Factor (unitless)	1.8	2.0–3.3
Minimum Self-Cleaning Velocity	Not typically used	0.5–0.6 m/s
Maximum Velocity	4 m/s	3–6 m/s
Minimum Tractive Tension[b]	0.1 kg/m^2 or 1 Pa	Not typically used
Minimum Flow Depth	0.20 x diameter	0.20 x diameter
Maximum Flow Depth	0.75 x diameter	0.75 x diameter
Minimum Design Flow	100–120 L/day/person	1500 L/day/person
Minimum Depth of Sewer	0.60–1.5 m	1.8 m
Minimum Depth of House Connection	0.4 m	0.8 m
Minimum Diameter	100 mm (house connections and block sewers) 150 mm (block collectors and trunk sewers)	150–200 mm
Minimum Slope	0.5%–0.6% (0.005–0.006 m/m)	1.0%–1.4% (0.01–0.014 m/m)
Maximum Manhole Spacing	(c)	100–180 m
Minimum Manhole Diameter	0.6–0.9 m	1.5 m
Typical Number of Homes per Collective Sewer or Street Lateral	10–60 homes for 100 mm diameter at min. slope and min. tractive tension	20 homes for 100 mm diameter at min. slope and min. velocity
Maximum Length of Pipe per Collective Sewer	400 m for 100 mm diameter at min. slope	Not typically used

Sources: Bakalian et al., 1994; Mara and Guimarães, 1999; WPCF, 1982; Sinnatamby, 1990, 147–48; Informant 76, CAERN social worker, interview by author, 11 April 1995, Natal; and Informant 77, CAERN civil engineer, interview by author, 25 May 1995, Natal.

a. The Manning formula is used in both condominial and conventional sewer design.

b. Minimum tractive tension is also known as minimum tractive force or critical boundary shear stress.

c. Fewer manholes are used in condominial sewer systems; most manholes are replaced by cleanout boxes (also known as inspection chambers).

d. m=meters; m^2=square meters; s=seconds; kg=kilograms; L=liters; mm=millimeters, Pa=Pascal.

resident installs a conventional house connection to the trunk sewer it is simply a matter of connecting their individual house to the existing sewer pipe. Existing neighborhoods can be retrofitted with conventional sewers that are installed in public streets to allow direct access by each and every home. An existing neighborhood also can be retrofitted with a condominial sewer installed on private property that collects sewage from groups of homes before discharging to the public sewer in the street.

Materials

Condominial sewers are typically made of either small diameter, inexpensive polyvinyl-chloride (PVC) or unvitrified clay pipe. Clay pipes are generally prone to more installation problems because they are manufactured in short sections (in 70-90 centimeter lengths for 100 millimeter diameter pipe[49]) and are subject to cracking and chipping at the joints. However, because of its durability and resistance to corrosion, clay pipe is the most commonly used condominial sewer construction material. Clay pipe is best used in areas with well-drained sandy soils and a low water table. In areas with poorly-drained soils and a high water table, PVC pipe offers a better alternative because it is manufactured in longer sections (in 6 meter lengths for 100 millimeter diameter pipe[50]) and has fewer joints and tighter joint connections, thereby minimizing the problems of infiltration and inflow.[51] Clay pipe is less expensive to buy and more durable than PVC pipes, but clay pipe is usually more expensive to install than PVC pipe. The short lengths of clay pipe generate more joints and more opportunities for error in laying the short lengths of pipe at a constant slope. Nevertheless, the total cost (purchase price plus installation cost) of PVC pipe tends to exceed the total cost of clay pipe,[52] and so clay pipe is more commonly used for condominial sewers. For house connections however, residents usually choose PVC because of its availability and ease of use. Both PVC and clay pipes have been used in Brazil. Photo 2-1 shows typical condominial sewer construction materials used in the Northeast region of the country. Photo 2-2 shows a typical household cleanout box installed in a backyard condominial sewer.

Closing Remarks for Chapter 2

This chapter introduced and summarized the wide-ranging reforms that were enacted in Brazil from the 1980s through the 1990s. The transition to democracy was summarized with special emphasis on the resulting decentralization of government in general and of the water and sanitation sector in particular. Corresponding with these national and state level reforms was Brazil's sanitation movement, a social movement of grassroots actors in solidarity with professional health care and environmental actors. These developments set the stage for a particular group of activist engineers in the Northeast region of the country to develop the technological innovation needed to expand access to sanitation service. Poor residents, influenced by the sanitation movement and the new democracy that seemed to welcome their involvement in public decision-making, were now organizing around demands for basic infrastructure services. The activist engineers responded and began to grasp not only the technical challenges of expanding sewer service to the poor, but also the social and financial challenges. Through research trials at the Universidade Federal do Rio Grande do Norte they developed a locally appropriate sanitation technology, and through the 1980s and early 1990s they experimented with various ways of implementing the new technology in actual neighborhoods. The next chapter introduces two urban settings in which the earliest innovations took place: Natal and Recife, Brazil.

See photo 2-1 in photospread at the end of this chapter.

See photo 2-2 in photospread at the end of this chapter.

Notes

1. Robert Gay, "Neighborhood Associations and Political Change in Rio de Janeiro," *Latin American Research Review* 25, no. 1 (1990): 102–18.

2. The BNH was reconstituted as the Federal Bank of Brazil (*Caixa Econômica Federal*, or CEF) in 1986.

3. Antonio Carlos Parlatore. *Privatization of the Water Utility Sector in Brazil* n.d. http://www.bndes.gov.br/english/studies/ensa/0-8.pdf (2003), 4.

4. Many of the original condominial sewer projects in Brazil were PLANASA/BNH-funded projects in which the World Bank provided a portion of the funds.

5. Ricardo Toledo Silva, "Urban Reconstruction and Institutional Reshaping in Brazil," in *The Challenge of Sustainable Cities: Neoliberalism and Urban Strategies in Developing Countries*, eds. Rod Burgess, Marisa Carmona, and Theo Kolstee (London and New Jersey: Zed Books, 1997), 26.

6. Tova Maria Solo, Eduardo Perez, and Steven Joyce. "Constraints in Providing Water and Sanitation Services to the Urban Poor," *Water Sanitation and Hygiene Report* 85 (Washington, DC: U.S. Agency for International Development, 1993).

7. Antonio Carlos Parlatore. *Privatization of the Water Utility Sector in Brazil*, 4–5.

8. David Samuels, "Reinventing Local Government? Municipalities and Intergovernmental Relations in Democratic Brazil," in *Democratic Brazil: Actors, Institutions, and Processes*, eds. Peter R. Kingstone and Timothy J. Power (Pittsburgh, PA: University of Pittsburgh Press, 2000), 82–83, 93.

9. Informant 120, URBANA civil engineer, interview by author, 25 May 1995, Natal, transcript.

10. Silvia Gerschman, "The Role of Social Movements in the Formulation of Health Policy in Brazil" (paper presented at Stanford University Center for Latin American Studies, Stanford, CA, March 3, 1993).

11. Scott Mainwaring, "Grassroots Popular Movements and the Struggle for Democracy: Nova Iguacu," in *Democratizing Brazil: Problems of Transition and Consolidation*, ed. Alfred Stepan (New York and Oxford: Oxford University Press, 1989), 199; and Scott

Mainwaring, "Grassroots Popular Movements, Identity, and Democratization in Brazil," *Kellogg Institute for International Studies Working Paper* 84 (Notre Dame, IN: University of Notre Dame, 1986).

12. Renato Raul Boschi. "The Art of Associating: Social Movements, The Middle Class, and Grassroots Politics in Urban Brazil," Final Report (New York: Tinker Foundation, 1984).

13. Their critique of the appropriateness of conventional sewer technology did not question the principal of waterborne sewerage itself, therefore keeping the critique within existing boundaries.

14. Boschi, "The Art of Associating: Social Movements, The Middle Class, and Grassroots Politics in Urban Brazil."

15. Gabrielle Watson. "Water and Sanitation in Sao Paulo, Brazil: Successful Strategies for Service Provision in Low-Income Communities," Master's thesis (Cambridge, MA: Massachusetts Institute of Technology, 1992).

16. Watson, "Water and Sanitation in Sao Paulo, Brazil."

17. Gay, "Neighborhood Associations and Political Change in Rio de Janeiro."

18. Gay, "Neighborhood Associations and Political Change in Rio de Janeiro."

19. Watson, "Water and Sanitation in Sao Paulo, Brazil."

20. Scott Mainwaring, "Grassroots Popular Movements and the Struggle for Democracy: Nova Iguacu," 188.

21. Scott Mainwaring, *Rethinking Party Systems in the Third Wave of Democratization: The Case of Brazil* (Stanford, CA: Stanford University Press, 1999), 90.

22. Gay, "Neighborhood Associations and Political Change in Rio de Janeiro."

23. Gay, "Neighborhood Associations and Political Change in Rio de Janeiro," 116.

24. Mainwaring, "Grassroots Popular Movements and the Struggle for Democracy: Nova Iguacu," 195; and Mainwaring, "Grassroots Popular Movements, Identity, and Democratization in Brazil," 27.

25. Boschi, "The Art of Associating: Social Movements, The Middle Class, and Grassroots Politics in Urban Brazil."

26. World Bank, *World Development Report 1994: Infrastructure for Development* (Washington, DC: Oxford University Press, 1994); and Albert Wright, "Toward a Strategic Sanitation Approach: Improving the Sustainability of Urban Sanitation in Developing Countries," (Washington, DC: The World Bank, 1997).

27. Deepa Narayan, "The Contribution of People's Participation: Evidence from 121 Rural Water Supply Projects," *UNDP-World Bank Water and Sanitation Program and Social Policy and Resettlement* (internal working document) (Washington, DC: World Bank, 1994); Philip R. Gerson, "Popular Participation in Economic Theory and Practice," *Human Resources Development and Operations Policy Working Paper* 18 (internal working paper) (Washington, DC: World Bank, 1993); and Wright, "Toward a Strategic Sanitation Approach: Improving the Sustainability of Urban Sanitation in Developing Countries," 9.

28. David C. Korten, "Community Organization and Rural Development: A Learning Process Approach," *Public Administration Review* 40 (1980): 480–511.

29. Korten, "Community Organization and Rural Development: A Learning Process Approach."

30. Informant 89, CAERN senior maintenance technician, interview by author, 19 May 1995, Natal, transcript.

31. José Carlos Melo, interview with author, January 2006, Recife, transcript.

32. Personal communication with Yves Cabannes, 2005, Cambridge, MA.

33. Solids-free sewers, known as "dreno" systems in Recife (where they were installed by COMPESA, the state water and sanitation agency), connect homes to an existing storm drain system, which may ultimately lead to a low-level treatment system (such as a stabilization pond), or which may discharge solids-free wastewater (or, in cases of cross connection and improperly maintained septic tanks, raw sewage) to a local water body.

34. Informant 89, CAERN senior maintenance technician, interview with author, 19 May 1995, Natal, transcript; and Informant 94, CAERN maintenance technician, interview with author, 19 May 1995, Natal, transcript.

35. Although the use of survey instruments is common engineering practice in the United States, they were not used consistently in Brazil at the time of the early condominial sewer projects.

36. Informant 75, CAERN senior civil engineer and sewer construction coordinator, interview with author, 23 May 1995, Natal, transcript.

37. Gehan Sinnatamby, "Low Cost Sanitation Systems for Urban Peripheral Areas in Northeast Brazil," Ph.D. dissertation (Leeds, UK: The University of Leeds, 1983).

38. The specific word for "sewer" used by lay Brazilians was as ambiguous as the sanitation situation of poor residents. The Portuguese word *rede de esgoto* means sewerage system. However, everyday people in the Northeast did not necessarily use or understand this meaning of the word in the early days of condominial sewerage. To everyday people, a *rede de esgoto* can also mean any manner of transporting wastewater (*esgoto*) through a network (*rede*), including either a sewer system or a network of street gutters, open ditches, or storm drains. The word *saneamento*, meaning sanitation, is commonly used to refer to water supply and sanitation collectively (as in *Companhia Pernambucana de Saneamento*, or the Water and Sanitation Company of Pernambuco), rather than to a specific system.

39. Eventually the technology would primarily become known as condominial sewers.

40. In this early period, the participatory development discourse had not yet realized the dominant position it would eventually achieve nor was the participation component being highlighted within the discourses of condominial sewers (which at the time were known by several other names as well). Therefore, it would be premature to apply the term participatory sanitation to the new sewer technology that was emerging. At this stage, proponents emphasized the new design criteria and lower costs in an attempt to differentiate condominial sewers from conventional sewers within an existing engineering framework that did not include participation.

41. Outstanding condominial sewer engineering texts have been written by Duncan Mara, *Low-Cost Urban Sanitation* (Chichester: John Wiley and Sons, 1996), and Gehan Sinnatamby, "Low Cost Sanitation," in *The Poor Die Young: Housing and Health in Third World Cities*, eds. Sandy Cairncross, Jorge E. Hardoy, and David Satterthwaite (London: Earthscan Publications, 1990).

42. It is very difficult to estimate the true cost of installed condominial sewer projects in Brazil because many of the projects were installed during an era of severe inflation. Brazil has experienced some of the highest inflation of any country, with inflation rates as high as 2,489 percent in 1993 (see Scott Mainwaring, *Rethinking Party Systems in the Third Wave of Democratization: The Case of Brazil*, 90). From 1985 to 1994, the average inflation rate in Brazil was 1,018 percent (Mainwaring, *Rethinking Party* Systems, 90). During this time, the price of a project would be re-calculated each month because the value of the Brazilian dollar was constantly changing, and by the end of a

typical project no one really knew its true cost. Heavy government subsidization of condominial sewer materials and monthly fees further complicates the estimation of true costs.

43. Abel Mejia, L. C. Tavares, Alexander Bakalian, and Vijay Jagannathan, "Water and Sanitation Services for the Urban Poor in Brazil: The PROSANEAR Approach," *World Bank Infrastructure Notes-Water and Sanitation* SW9 (Washington, DC: World Bank, 1993). Based on 4.39 people per household for the project areas studied (Instituto Brasileiro de Geografia e Estatística, 1991), the reported range of $48 to $123 in per capita cost is equivalent to a range of $211 to $540 per connection (in 1993 U.S. dollars).

44. Alexander Bakalian, Albert Wright, Richard Otis, and José M. Azevedo-Netto, *Simplified Sewerage: Design Guidelines* (Washington, DC: The World Bank, 1994) José M. Azevedo-Netto, "Innovative and Low Cost Technologies Utilized in Sewerage," *Environmental Health Program Technical Series* 29 (Washington, DC: Pan American Health Organization and World Health Organization, 1992), 48; World Bank, *World Development Report 1992: Development and the Environment* (Washington, DC: Oxford University Press, 1992), 108; Albert M. Wright and Alexander E. Bakalian, "Intermediate Sanitation: Cost Efficient Sewerage," *World Bank Infrastructure Notes-Water and Sanitation* SW-4 (Washington, DC: World Bank, 1990); and Carlos Alberto dos Santos and Adejalmo Figueiredo Gazen, "Estudo Comparativo Entre Redes Coletoras de Esgotos do Tipo Convencional e Não Convencional," Convenio ASFAMAS-PVC e ABIVINILA, Artigo Tecnico, Setembro de 1987: 5.

45. Informant 12, COMPESA engineer, interview by author, 10 March 1995, Recife, transcript.

46. Sinnatamby, "Low Cost Sanitation," 148.

47. Bakalian et al., *Simplified Sewerage: Design Guidelines*, 23.

48. Bakalian et al., *Simplified Sewerage: Design Guidelines*, 23; and Sinnatamby, "Low Cost Sanitation," 148.

49. Informant 100, president of an engineering company, interview by author, 19 March 1995, Recife, transcript.

50. Informant 100, president of an engineering company, interview by author, 19 March 1995, Recife, transcript.

51. As defined by Robert Corbitt, *Standard Handbook of Environmental Engineering* (New York: McGraw-Hill, 1990), 6, 62, infiltration is "the groundwater which leaks into the sewer system generally through deteriorated and/or defective pipes, joints, connections, and manholes. . . . Inflow is the storm water which directly enters the sewer system after rainfall from such sources as flooded manhole covers, yard and roof drain connections, and cross-connections with a storm sewer."

52. Informant 100, president of an engineering company, interview by author, 19 March 1995, Recife, transcript.

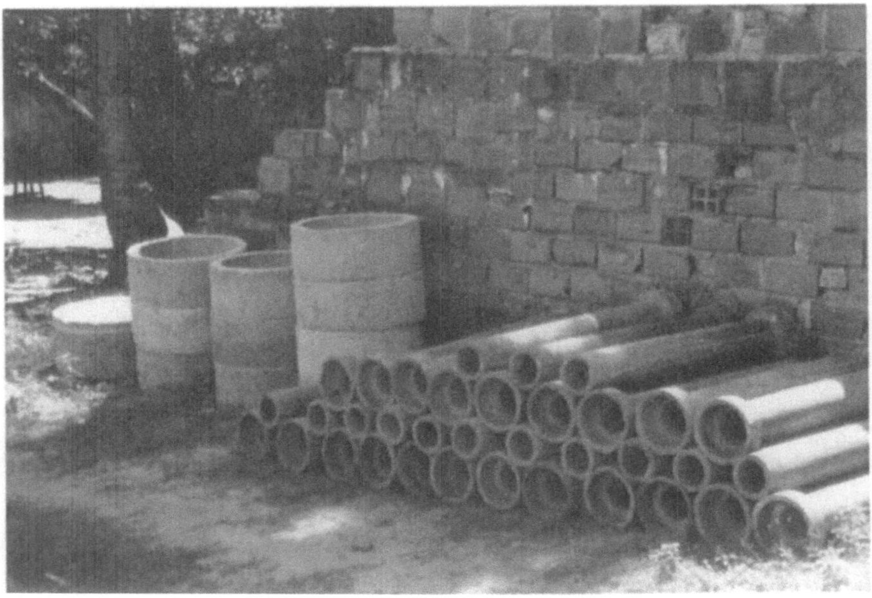

Photo 2-1. Typical condominial sewer construction materials: clay pipes and concrete cleanout boxes. (Source: Photograph taken by the author, 1995).

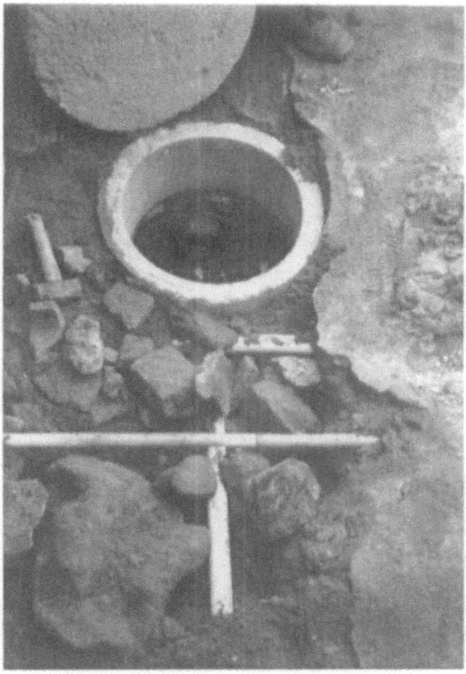

Photo 2-2. Typical installed cleanout box for a backyard condominial sewer system in Brazil. (Source: Photograph taken by the author, 1995).

Chapter 3
Situating Services in Two Brazilian Cities

While Brazil is often discussed in terms of its past peripheral position in the global economy and more recently in terms of its status as a newly industrialized country (as of 2011), understanding the reproduction and maintenance of poverty in Brazil requires within-country analysis. To appreciate Brazil's struggle to address the sanitation dimension of its poverty problem, one must investigate the local conditions that created the innovation locally known as *condominial sewerage*. The promise of participatory development expressed in chapter 1 and the water and sanitation reforms presented in chapter 2 came to life at the local level in Brazilian cities. This chapter delves deeper into these local conditions by introducing the sanitation situations of the first two cities to experiment with condominial sewerage.

The Northeast capital cities of Natal and Recife offer contrasting contexts for observing the emergence of condominial sewerage. The urban geography and living conditions of these two local settings are described, followed by an explanation of the governance structures in which sanitation services were delivered. The chapter also presents new methods for observing and measuring citizen involvement and project outcome. These methods form the basis of comparison for projects that arose in different local settings, and will be used in the comparative case analysis that is presented in subsequent chapters.

Social Exclusion in Brazil

In order to survive, impoverished people often settle on the most marginal lands and construct their own shelters. These shantytowns and squatter settlements, known in Brazil as *favelas,* are created because access to housing and infrastructure services is differentiated on the basis of capital.[1] Although the institutions that reproduce poverty are not limited to Brazilian society, they have certainly flourished there as demonstrated by the extremes of poverty endured by generations of Brazilians. Poverty is the fundamental feature of the two study areas.

Favelas are characterized by high population densities, low-income levels, lack of legal land tenure, and lack of formal water, sanitation, electricity, and other infrastructure services.[2] Favelas first appeared in Rio de Janeiro in the late 1890s. Squatter settlements continued to grow in all major Brazilian cities, especially during the post-war population explosion of the 1940s.[3] From the late 1960s to the early 1980s, one third of Rio de Janeiro's population lived in favelas.[4] In 1993, 60 million people out of a total Brazilian population of 150 million lived in favelas, and 12 million had no residence.[5] Official Brazilian policy in the decades following World War II was to prevent new favelas and to eliminate old ones. But it was only after the military takeover in 1964 that the Brazilian government could begin to muster the power and resources to implement these goals.[6] One result was that, in 1973, the city of Rio de Janeiro planned to eliminate all of its favelas within ten years.[7] Governments of Brazil had always exhibited strong authoritarian tendencies, and these tendencies were expressed to their fullest in the two-decade reign of Brazil's repressive military government from 1964 to 1984. The repressive climate of this era included the prohibition of individual freedoms, "disappearances," the use of torture, and favela-eradication programs. The military regime also guided Brazil toward unprecedented economic growth, culminating in the so-called economic miracle of 1968-1974. Unfortunately, this economic boom led to increasing income concentration and poverty,[8] and it was soon followed by sharp economic decline, hyperinflation, and massive foreign debt in the 1980s.

Brazil's institutions have excelled in creating and reproducing social and economic exclusion. Both the richest and poorest people of Latin America live in Brazil. In the early 1990s, the income of the 40th percentile of poorest families in Brazil was lower than the equivalent percentile of any other country, and the income of the 20th percentile of richest families in Brazil was higher than the equivalent percentile of any other country.[9] In 1980, 50 percent of the poorest people in Brazil earned only 13 percent of the total income, while 46 percent of the total income went to the richest 10 percent of Brazilians.[10] In 2001, approximately 62 percent of the Brazilian population had an income of two minimum salaries or less[11] (in 2001, two minimum salaries was approximately R$360,[12] the equivalent of about US$5.17 per day).[13] The extreme maldistribution of land ownership was an important factor in reproducing inequitable distribution of and exclusion from basic resources and services.[14] Inequality in Brazil, as measured by a GINI index of 59.3 in 2001, is consistently "in the highest range of inequality" of all countries in the world.[15]

Brazil's regional disparities worsened with the increasing urbanization and industrialization of the twentieth century. Brazilians in the Southeast states (including Sao Paulo) experienced the highest average incomes and the lowest relative level of inequality, while the Northeast region—the historic center of Brazil's slave economy—continued to have the highest degree of inequality and the lowest average incomes.[16] In the 1970s, inequality decreased and average family incomes increased in the Southeast region, but in the Northeast inequality worsened and average family incomes dropped during the same period.[17] The economic disparities between the Northeast region and the rest of Brazil are also reflected in the statistics on access to water and sanitation. Northeast citizens are disproportionately excluded from basic services such as water supply and sanitation. In 1999, the percentage of Northeastern households with access to piped water (59 percent) and sewers (23 percent) was far less than the average household in Brazil, in which 76 percent had piped water and 53 percent had a sewer system.[18] Because of these great regional imbalances, countrywide generalizations tend to be inaccurate for Brazil.

In the late 1980s, over 70 percent of Brazil's population lived in urban areas, where the proliferation of favelas was common.[19] Much of this urbanization was the result of mass migrations of the landless poor from rural areas into the cities. Urban population growth without corresponding increases in urban services resulted in poor public health and degraded urban environments. The consequences of exclusion from affordable sanitation services resulted in discharges of raw sewage into open ditches (*valas negras*) in favelas and low-income areas, and a higher risk of death from sanitation-related diseases such as cholera, typhoid, diarrhea, and dysentery.[20]

The extent to which sanitation is inadequate directly affects public health and economic productivity. Regarding the former, diseases can quickly reach epidemic proportions in the unsanitary conditions of most high-density urban neighborhoods and favelas. For example, cholera spread rapidly throughout Latin America in the early 1990s. Cholera first reached epidemic levels in Peru and then spread to the Northeast region of Brazil. Subsequently, the disease spread to Brazil's South and Southeast regions. By 1994, a total of 378,488 people had been stricken with cholera throughout Latin America, with 150,000 cases and 1,700 deaths reported in Brazil.[21] Favela residents were most vulnerable to epidemics such as these, in addition to the chronic endemic diseases that disproportionately affected poor neighborhoods. Sanitation-related health problems resulting from the lack of water supply and sanitary sewerage prevent people from participating in income-generating activities that could contribute to their own welfare and to society.[22] Clearly, basic water and sanitation services are investments in both public health and economic productivity.

Low-cost technologies such as condominial sewers are particularly appropriate for poor regions such as the Northeast region of Brazil which, for reasons already cited, have been excluded from the benefits of development. Compared with Brazil's other regions, experience with condominial sewers in the Northeast has been the most widespread and the most successful,[23] so this geographic region was the most fruitful area to study. Familiarity with local conditions is essential to an understanding of project success and failure. The remainder of this chapter is dedicated to describing the relevant conditions in Brazil's Northeast region that necessitated and nurtured the condominial sewer movement.

The Target Areas of Study

The Northeast region of Brazil (one of five geographic regions) historically has been the poorest and least developed geographic area in the country. It is the location of historic slavery in Brazil, and the location of Brazil's first national capital: Recife. The Northeast region represents 27.5 percent of Brazil's land area, 12 percent of the gross domestic product, and 16 percent of Brazil's population,[24] but it remains economically depressed compared to the rest of Brazil. The region is characterized by low economic growth, high poverty, frequent droughts, and semi-feudal relations between powerful landholders and rural citizens. Poverty predominates as a consequence of the history of colonialism, slavery, and inequitable land ownership. A class of Brazilian oligarchs holds most of the land in huge, often fallow, plots (*latifundias*) greater than 1,000 hectares.[25] According to Sauer, "the country has one of the world's most perverse and highly concentrated landholding structures, with a Gini index near 0.9—nearly total concentration—as a result of its segregationist agriculture and land-tenure system."[26] The ten-year average monthly income per person in the Northeast (for the decade ending in 1999) was only 1.2 minimum salaries (just slightly above the poverty line); the average among the other regions of Brazil for the same decade was 2.4 minimum salaries.[27]

Table 3-1 provides an assessment of income categories for urban households in the Northeast region of Brazil from data on the distribution of income in 2000. Based on the World Bank's approach, households with incomes of two minimum salaries or less are considered living in poverty, and households with incomes of one minimum salary or less are considered living in extreme poverty.[28] "Low" incomes in Brazil are locally perceived to be in the range of two to five minimum salaries per household, "middle" incomes range from five to eight minimum salaries per household, and "high" incomes are greater than eight minimum salaries per household.[29] Table 3-1 reveals that in 2000 approximately 65 percent of Northeast urban households were poor, indigent, or had no income; and that 30 percent of households reported no income or less than one minimum salary per household. The income categories defined in Table 3-1 will be referred to in the remainder of this book.

Two coastal cities in the Northeast—Recife (capital of the state of Pernambuco) and Natal (capital of the state of Rio Grande do Norte)—are the birthplace of condominial sewers. Both cities began implementing condominial sewers in the early 1980s. By 1994, each city had installed well over ten thousand condominial sewer connections. Recife and Natal are each over 460 years old, but their different historical and political-economic conditions resulted in different patterns of condominial sewer implementation and in different outcomes. Natal's urbanization and population growth have primarily developed since World War II, so the city has a more modern appearance than Recife. Most of Recife's growth and development took place hundreds of years ago. Recife has a class of very wealthy people as a result of its past agricultural economies in sugar cane, coffee, cotton, and tobacco; the international port; and the city's well-developed industrial sector. The jobs resulting from this wealth combined with desperate rural circumstances have historically attracted the rural poor to emigrate from the interior and from other states in the Northeast region to Recife. Natal does not have this level of old wealth, but it still has poverty. Many of Natal's poorest people live in favelas on the periphery of the city, while in Recife the poor live within the city itself as well as on the urban fringe. Although in 1999-2000 the population of Recife (1.4 million) was approximately twice that of Natal (0.71 million), more of Recife's households lived in poverty. For example, 29.1 percent of Recife's households were located in favelas, and 6.83 percent of Natal's households were located in favelas.[30]

Compared to Natal, Recife is surrounded by a larger metropolitan community that includes the cities of Olinda and Jaboatao. Recife is larger in land area and population, and is more economically developed than Natal. During the time period of this study, Recife was a large city while Natal grew from a medium-sized city to a large city.[31] From 1980 to 2010, Natal's population increased at a higher rate than Recife's population (113 percent in Natal, 30 percent in Recife). An average of 24 percent of the Rio Grando do Norte state population resided in the capital city of Natal, and 18 percent of the Pernambuco state population resided in Recife. City, state, and nationwide population figures for the study period are summarized in Table 3-2. In 2000, Natal had an average population density of 4,219 people/square kilometer compared to 6,536 in Recife, indicating Natal was about two-thirds as dense as Recife.[32]

Like Recife, Natal is built on a river floodplain; however, Natal does not have the flat topography, the high water table, and the poor soil conditions of Recife. Natal also has a drier climate than Recife. Consequently, Natal's drainage problems are not nearly on the scale of the drainage problems in Recife. In both cities, but in Recife especially, interconnections between storm drains and sanitary sewers result in a great volume of untreated sewage. Both Natal and Recife suffer from a severe shortage of sewage treatment capacity, and both cities treat only a paltry percentage of the total sewage collected. Both cities exhibit a pattern in which the better performing sewer systems tend to be located in neighborhoods with higher average incomes, and the worst performing projects tend to be located in the poorer neighborhoods; however, there are some important exceptions to this pattern which will be discussed in a later chapter. With regard to sewer expansion from the late 1980s to the mid 1990s, sewer connections (conventional and condominial) in Natal grew by 18 percent while sewer connections in Recife grew by 11 percent overall.[33]

With respect to the local environments for implementing condominial sewer projects, statements from condominial sewer practitioners in both cities indicate that they perceived differences between the two cities. Two sewer agency staff members in Natal reported that Recife was "more politically advanced" than Natal in terms of people recognizing their citizenship rights, mobilizing to meet the basic needs of their communities, and joining political parties.[34] An engineer

Table 3-1. Estimates of household income using average monthly income per household, in minimum salaries, for urban households in the Northeast region of Brazil in 2000.

Income per Household in Minimum Salaries per Month	No. of Households in 2000	Percent of Total Households[a]	Estimated Household Income Level[b]
No income	758,514	8.37%	no income
Up to 1	1,922,329	21.21%	indigent[c]
From 1 to 3	3,194,140	35.25%	poor[c]
From 3 to 5	1,262,249	13.93%	low income
From 5 to 10	1,046,545	11.55%	middle income[d]
More than 10	878,806	9.70%	high income

Source: IBGE Censo Demográfico, http://www.ibge.gov.br/home/estatistica/populacao/censo2000/trabalho_rendimento/tabela_regioes.shtm?c=2, 2000.

a. These calculations use data from IBGE.

b. This characterization of income level was informed by the work of Rocha (1997) and World Bank (2003). The poverty line in Brazil is often difficult to determine. The cost of a "food basket" (*cesta básica*) of basic foodstuffs for one month is typically set as the poverty line (Power and Roberts, 2000, 248), however, several other methods for determining the poverty line are also in use (Rocha, 1997, 4). A *cesta básica* for a family of four cost 2.37 minimum salaries in Natal as of April 2001 (Escoda et al, 2001, 5).

c. In Brazil, indigent and poor people often live in shantytowns or squatter settlements called *favelas*, thus the people are commonly referred to as *favelados*. People who inhabited favelas in Recife in the early 1980s earned up to 3 minimum salaries per household, but the great majority of Recife's favela dwellers earned between 1 and 2 minimum salaries per household (Prefeitura da Cidade do Recife, 1983, 4).

d. The middle income category can be further divided into three subcategories: 1) lower middle income (more than 5 up to 6 minimum salaries), middle middle income (more than 6 up to 9 minimum salaries), and upper middle income (more than 9 up to 10 minimum salaries).

Table 3-2. Population growth from 1980 to 2010, in millions of people.

Year	Brazil	Pernambuco	Recife	Rio Grande do Norte	Natal
1980	121.286	6.142	1.184	1.898	0.3766
1991	151.152	7.128	1.298	2.416	0.6069
1996	161.365	7.399	1.346	2.559	0.6560
2000	172.860	7.918	1.422	2.777	0.7095
2005	184.389	8.421	1.501	3.006	0.7899
2010	190.733	8.796	1.538	3.168	0.8037

Source: Populstat, 1999/2003 and 1999/2006; IBGE, 2010; IBGE PNAD 2005; and Wikimapia. (Note: Natal's 2006 population is used for 2005).

in Recife reported that Natal was "more evolved" than Recife in terms of condominial sewer implementation.[35] In later chapters, I give an account of specific projects and programs that reveals why these statements reflect important differences between Recife and Natal, differences that had direct effects on the success and failure of condominial sewerage.

Urban Geography and Infrastructure

What geographic features of the two cities affected the available options for sanitation development? In this brief sub-section, I present the general geographic and infrastructure conditions of each city at the mid-point of the study period (ca. 1995).

Recife[36]

Recife was built in the coastal floodplain of the Capibaribe, the Tejipio, and the Beberibe rivers (i.e., *Rio Capibaribe, Rio Tejipio,* and *Rio Beberibe*). When the Dutch ruled the city in the 1600s, they installed a system of canals to drain the city of excess water. This system has been updated and expanded over the years to form a ninety-two-kilometer-long network of sixty-six canals. The drainage problem in Recife has profound implications for sanitation. A relatively high water table, a generally flat topography, and poorly drained soils increase the difficulty of collecting, transporting, and discharging wastewater

In the mid 1990s, the Recife city government (*Prefeitura da Cidade do Recife*, or PCR) adopted a sanitation master plan (*Plano Estruturador de Esgotamento Sanitário do Recife*) that mandated the use of condominial sewers in all future planned increases in sewer coverage. By legitimizing the condominial option, this plan was an attempt to extend service to previously excluded segments of the population. By December 1994, an estimated 24 percent of the Recife population (and 18 percent of the metropolitan region population) was connected to the public sewer system (conventional and condominial), and the remaining 76 percent of the population discharged sewage into onsite systems (i.e., leach pits, cesspools, or septic tanks), storm drain connections, street gutters, or open ditches. Regardless of which sewage collection method was used, most collected sewage was ultimately discharged untreated to rivers and canals that flow to the ocean.

Recife is located in the state of Pernambuco. Like other states in Brazil, Pernambuco is divided into counties (*municipios*), cities, political-administrative regions (*regiões politico-administrativos*, or RPAs), and neighborhoods (*localidades* or *bairros*). The State Water and Sanitation Agency of Pernambuco (*Companhia Pernambucana de Saneamento*, or COMPESA) further divided the state into water supply districts (*escritórios locais*, or *elos*), which were typically larger than a neighborhood, except in cases where a very large neighborhood made up an entire "elo." These *elos* were purely administrative, and they did not necessarily correspond to watersheds or drainage basin boundaries.

As of 1995 Recife had seven water districts (*elos*), three regional sewer divisions, and 98 sewer basins, the boundaries of which corresponded neither to each other nor to the county, city, RPA, or neighborhood boundaries. In addition to these boundaries, poor areas were further classified as special economic zones (*zeis*). The Recife metropolitan area (which in 1995 contained about 3 million people) had approximately 950 km of sewer pipe and three regional wastewater treatment plants, each serving a sewer division. The Cabanga and Peixinhos regional treatment plants are located in the city of Recife, and the Janga regional treatment plant is located in the nearby city of Olinda. There were eighty-three pump stations and twenty-eight small local treatment plants in the Recife Metropolitan Region (RMR).

Most of Recife's public sewer system was interconnected with the storm drain and canal systems, and cross-contamination was ubiquitous. Conventional sewers in Recife were required to have overflow (*extravassor*) pipes to route sewer overflows into storm drain canals, storm drain pipes, or rivers. These overflow pipes were employed in the frequent case of pump station loss due to a power outage or maintenance. Multiple overflow pipes were often installed at various heights, so large volumes of sewage typically ended up in the storm drain system and in local surface waters.

Natal[37]

Natal is a coastal city built in the floodplain of the Potengi River (i.e., *Rio Potengi*) in the state of Rio Grande do Norte. Natal's conventional sewer infrastructure was built by the U.S. military during World War II. The United States, an ally of Brazil, stationed its military base in Natal because it was the shortest distance from the Americas to the African front. Brazil benefited in several ways, one of which was the installation of conventional sewers in Natal by the U.S. military. The conventional sewer system built in the 1940s was well-made using conservative sewer system design criteria that called for large, deep vitrified ceramic and concrete pipes (up to nine meters deep in some places) and full-size concrete manholes laid in the middle of paved streets.

Natal's conventional sewer system begins in the Ribeira district and flows through the central city. In 1967, Natal expanded the conventional sewer system, but by 1995 Natal still had only one operating stabilization pond to treat the collected sewage. Additional treatment capacity was still in the planning stages.

The Sanitation Circumstances of Residents

I obtained firsthand accounts of the sanitation situations in which people lived and a range of citizen viewpoints by interviewing hundreds of households and dozens of condominial sewer practitioners who worked in communities in Recife and Natal. The information presented below focuses on the time period of the early 1980s through the mid-1990s, the period when condominial sewers were first being developed. The following text illustrates how people excluded from conventional sewer service managed their household wastewater prior to the advent of condominial sewers.

Recife

Because of the generally low rate of service provision in Recife during the early 1980s, it was customary for unserved residents to manage their sewage by using individual solutions. The most common individual solutions were onsite leach pits, onsite cesspools, onsite septic tanks, vacant areas, clandestine connections to storm drains, the "dreno" system (which sent septic tank effluent to storm drains),[38] and open ditches that transported sewage to street gutters, storm drains, rivers, or canals. When an onsite system stopped working, sewage either backed up onto the property and into the house of the resident, or it overflowed onto neighboring properties whose systems may have been working normally. In some cases, sewage even backed up into the houses of neighbors interconnected to a common collection pipe.

Community septic tanks tended to function better than onsite septic tanks because of better siting decisions and better maintenance. Onsite household septic tanks were usually installed in any convenient location determined by the homeowner, while the location of community septic tanks was determined by engineers. The "dreno" systems typically functioned well at first; however, if residents forgot to maintain their septic tank then solids ended up passing into the dreno pipes when the septic tank filled up. Some residents only cleaned out their septic tank when the sewage overflowed into the yard or into the house. In 1994-1995, the typical cost to a resident for cleaning out an onsite septic tank was R$200 per truckload (roughly US$200 at that time).[39] This was extremely expensive for a low-income individual, who typically earned about R$300 per month (roughly US$300 at that time), the equivalent of about four minimum salaries.

Residents who were satisfied with their individual sewage solutions typically did not feel the need to connect to and pay for a separate sewer system, and consequently they did not typically express a desire to further resolve sewage problems at the regional or citywide level. Once the sewage problem moved beyond most residents' individual lot or block, there was typically little willingness to participate or mobilize around sanitation issues.[40] On the other hand, Recife residents in the following circumstances expressed higher levels of demand for sewer infrastructure and tended to be more willing to mobilize around and participate in sewer solutions:[41]

- Residents whose only option was to discharge to open ditches (*valas negras*);
- Residents whose onsite septic tanks, leach pits, or cesspools did not function well (because of poor drainage, high water table, shoddy construction, or lack of funds to pay for pumping); and
- Residents who did not have other infrastructure or topographic conditions that effectively reduced the build-up of sewage on their property (such as storm drains, good topography, or pavement).

During the 1980s in Recife there were approximately one million unpaved streets in the city.[42] Consequently, most residents expressed a primary demand for pavement. It was commonly believed that pavement would simultaneously solve both the drainage problem and the sewage problem, because paved streets would improve the control of runoff and street gutters would collect and transport sewage away from homes.

Most residents in Recife had a basic understanding of how individual onsite wastewater solutions worked because they were familiar with them. But during the early 1980s, many residents were not familiar with condominial sewers. The technology was new and only a few condominial sewer systems had been installed. The following statements typify viewpoints expressed by practitioners about the public's level of familiarity with sewers at that time:[43]

> Residents don't know the difference between a storm drain and a condominial sewer, and when a storm drain exists they use it as a sewer.
>
> Sewers are a question of culture, and a sewer culture does not exist. People have televisions, stereos, and refrigerators, but not toilets.

Perhaps no other issue created more tension than the idea that condominial sewer users had to maintain their own systems. Many residents preferred and expected maintenance support from the sewer agency, even if they had signed an agreement accepting to take on responsibility for maintenance, as revealed in the following anonymous comments by residents:[44]

> A government agency already exists to provide this service.
>
> The government has better tools and equipment to do the job.
>
> I pay the sewer fee each month, which includes maintenance service.
>
> I tried to do it myself and gave up.
>
> Most of the problems are in the public part of the sewer.

Natal

Residents in Natal had a variety of different sanitation circumstances prior to receiving a condominial sewer. Affluent households with land typically had well-functioning septic tanks (*fossa sépticas*) connected to leach pits (*sumidouros*). Solids remained in the septic tank and solids-free wastewater flowed to the leach pit, where it seeped into the ground. Septic tank functioning was enhanced by the presence of the leach pit and by regular cleaning of the septic tank. In most affluent households, indoor plumbing fixtures (i.e., sinks, showers, toilets, and drains) were already piped to the household septic tank and leach pit, so if a condominial sewer was eventually installed, it was relatively easy to connect the sewer to the existing pipe. Affluent residents could afford high-quality construction of these house connections, and their neighborhoods tended to have adequate drainage infrastructure. These two circumstances ultimately contributed to the performance of any future condominial sewer, first because of the higher probability of good construction quality and second because of the lower tendency to connect rainwater to the sewer system, which caused system overflows.

Less affluent residents in Natal typically had a septic tank but lacked a leach pit. In this situation, the septic tank filled up sooner because it received both solid waste and wastewater. Less affluent residents could not always afford to have their septic tank cleaned out regularly. The price to clean out a septic tank in 1995 was less than one minimum salary, about R$55 to R$60 per month (roughly equivalent to US$55 to US$60 per month in March 1995), which included disposal of the septic sludge into the company's stabilization pond. This price was inexpensive compared to Recife where it cost on the order of R$200 (two minimum salaries) and where some companies discharged illegally to canals, storm drains, or vacant sites because they did not own adequate discharge locations.

Some low-income and poor residents used simple septic tanks whereby solids remained in the septic tank and an overflow pipe carried the wastewater to a storm drain or canal (this solution is comparable to the "dreno" system of Recife). Other low-income and poor residents in Natal employed simple septic tanks that connected only to their toilets. Sewage flowed into the septic tank, and all other household wastewaters (known as graywater) were collected in buckets and thrown into the street. This allowed the septic tank to function longer between cleanings, which was important because low-income and poor residents typically could not afford regular septic tank cleaning. Nevertheless, the sanitation situation of these residents (compared to more affluent residents) was often the worst in terms of public health. Also, it was a relatively difficult and expensive task to connect household fixtures if a condominial sewer was eventually installed, because only the toilet had been previously piped. These residents also could not typically afford high-quality construction. Instead of buying regular pipes, they might have bought half-pipes (open on top) to route solids-free wastewaters to the condominial sewer cleanout box. This solution reduced system capacity because it allowed rainwater to enter the sewer. When low-income and poor residents did install house connections to the sewer clean-out box, pieces of brick or concrete could enter the system and increase the possibility of future blockages. Low-income and poor residents typically could only afford to connect each household fixture to their condominial sewer one by one, and the process of connecting all fixtures often took months.[45]

Residents living in favelas and very poor areas typically did not fall into any of the four income groups previously described, and they were often left out of formal infrastructure expansion plans. Natal's state water and sanitation agency (*Companhia de Águas e Esgotos do Rio Grande do Norte*, or CAERN) did not include favelas in its initial condominial sewer programs during the period studied. As of 1995, CAERN had not implemented condominial sewers in any of Natal's favelas. Instead, the agency had implemented thousands of condominial sewer connections in low-income and poor (non-favela) areas of Natal. CAERN staff reported that they prioritized low-income and poor residents (and not favela residents) because of the health problems associated with discharging gray water into city streets. Many favela neighborhoods did not have streets or were defined as being outside formal city boundaries.

Formal Organizations for Delivering Sanitation Service

How did the cities of Recife and Natal organize to deliver sanitation services to previously excluded residents? During the early period of condominial sewer development, formal organizational structures had not yet been formed or solidified as institutions for delivering infrastructure services. The early approaches for organizing condominial sewers were experimental and were tied visibly to local political administrations. While the cities of Recife and Natal had institutionalized conventional sanitation at the state level—each having a state-owned water and sanitation company charged with implementing services—the organizations for condominial sewerage were significantly different in each city. These differences in city-level service organizations are described in the following subsections.

Condominial Sewer Organizations in Recife

Numerous local and state organizations were involved in condominial sewer implementation in Recife during the 1980 to 1995 period of condominial sewer development. The Pernambuco State Water and Sanitation Agency (COMPESA) and the Pernambuco State Housing Agency (*Companhia da Habitação*, or COHAB) each had roles in implementing the initial condominial sewer systems in addition to implementing conventional sewer systems, water supply systems, and housing projects. At the municipal level, the City of Recife Urban Planning Agency (*Empresa de Planejamento Urbano do Recife*, or URB) and the City of Recife Public Works Agency (*Empresa de Obras Públicas*, or OBRAS;[46] later renamed the Urban Cleanup Agency, *Empresa Municipal de Limpeza Urbana*, or EMLURB) were responsible for the planning, design, construction, and maintenance of the initial condominial sewers in Recife, as well as pavement, drainage, trash collection, street cleaning, and tree control services (but not conventional sewers).

COMPESA was responsible for the planning, design, construction, maintenance, and billing of water and sanitation infrastructure for the State of Pernambuco. COMPESA consisted of a president, five directorates, and various departments, such as the Metropolitan Sewer Department (*Gerência Metropolitana de Esgotos*, or GME), which maintained the regional sewer system, pump stations, and treatment plants of Recife. There were three sewer divisions in Recife—Peixinhos, Sul, and Cabanga—each with its own chief. On a day-to-day basis, the Division Chief decided which projects and which neighborhoods received maintenance service.

COMPESA's maintenance budget was typically very limited. During March of 1995, COMPESA had three sewer maintenance trucks and an operations and maintenance budget of only R$9000 per month (equivalent to about US$9000) for the entire Peixinhos sewer division.[47] According to COMPESA staff, maintaining the trucks was the biggest expense. Several informants from COMPESA reported that water supply was, "without a doubt," the top priority for both COMPESA and the public because there were still cities in Pernambuco without an adequate supply of water.[48] From 1980 to 1995, sewerage was the second priority for the agency. By 1995, COMPESA had not constructed any major sewer works for fifteen years; the agency had only installed a few small isolated projects.

In Recife, condominial sewer fees were charged as a percentage of the water bill. Residential water bills were determined either by the volume of water consumed (for metered households) or by a flat rate (for unmetered households).[49] In January 1995, the minimum water tariff (the rate charged to unmetered households) was R$2.60 per month (equivalent to US$2.60 per month at that time). Fees for condominial sewer service in Recife varied depending on the type of layout and by which agency implemented the project. In 1995, City agencies and COMPESA charged 40 percent of the household water bill for backyard and front yard condominial sewer layouts, 80 percent of the water bill for sidewalk condominial sewer layouts, 50 percent for dreno systems installed by COMPESA, and 100 percent for conventional sewers.[50] COHAB charged 80 percent of the household water bill for condominial sewers regardless of layout, and 100 percent for conventional sewers.[51] In January 1995, the minimum charge for a backyard condominial sewer was R$1.04 per month (equivalent to US$1.04 per month)[52] for an unmetered household. COMPESA issued colorful pamphlets to teach sewer system users how to carry out their ongoing maintenance responsibilities.[53] The content of one such pamphlet is presented in Table 3-3.

Condominial Sewer Organizations in Natal

Natal's sewer agency, the North Rio Grand State Water and Sanitation Agency (*Companhia de Águas e Esgotos do Rio Grande do Norte*, or CAERN) divided Natal into fifteen sewer basins and multiple water sectors. Sewer basins were bigger than water sectors and usually contained several water sectors. Sewer basins were hydrologically based, while water sectors were commercial divisions for billing, administration, and other purposes. CAERN organized sewer funding, planning, engineering, and construction based on the sewer basin unit (theoretically), so projects were known by their sewer basin name (e.g., Basin A, Basin B, Basin C, etc.), in addition to the name of the neighborhood served. A single sewer project may include more than one neighborhood or may serve only a fraction of a single neighborhood. During the implementation of a condominial sewer project, CAERN engineers designed projects around the sewer basin unit and CAERN participation staff (i.e., the engineers, social workers, and technicians who implemented CAERN's participation program) designed their participation programs around the smaller water sector unit. However, CAERN organized its complaint and repair records by neighborhood, not by sewer basin or water sector. Because CAERN often distributed scarce maintenance resources to satisfy the political objectives of the state governor, knowing which neighborhood was being served was important to the decision makers.[54]

Table 3-3. Instructions to users on sewer system maintenance responsibilities.

Step	Instructions
1	Each resident is responsible for maintaining the household connection to their property.
2	Verify the location of the blockage. Find out which cleanout box is downstream of the blocked one.
3	Open the cleanout box carefully in order not to break it. Obtain a thick wire with a wad of cloth tied to the end.
4	Remove the blocked material with a shovel. Be careful, it is contaminated.
5	Close up the cleanout box and seal it with cement, preventing the escape of odors and insects.
6	Show your neighbors the blocked material that caused the blockage.
7	Bury the material to prevent contact with people or animals.

Source: COMPESA (no date). Translated by author.

CAERN was led by a Directorate consisting of a president, an engineer, and an administrator, each appointed by the governor. CAERN was divided into three divisions: Projects (*Setor de Projetos*), Construction (*Setor de Obras*), and Operation (*Setor de Operação*). In May of 1994, staff of the Construction Division consisted of three engineers, one social scientist, three engineering technicians, one administrative technician, and sixteen student interns from the local sanitation vocational school.[55] The Projects Division was staffed with one engineer, four engineering technicians, and eight student interns.[56] In January 1995, CAERN took steps to decentralize its operation by extending its maintenance offices into the four administrative regions of the city to better serve its customers and to follow the nationwide decentralization of the sector.

CAERN's Directorate focused most of the agency's sewer maintenance resources (for Natal) on the sewage collection system, which included sewage pump stations, conventional sewers, and condominial sewers.[57] Few resources were applied to maintaining Natal's sewage treatment system, a centralized stabilization pond that provided the only form of treatment for sewage collected from the city. By 1995, CAERN's neglect of the treatment system was readily visible in the poor functioning of the plant.

CAERN charged a 40 percent monthly fee for backyard and front yard condominial sewer layouts (as a percentage of the water bill), an 80 percent fee for sidewalk condominial sewers, and a 100 percent fee for conventional sewers.[58] In 1994-1995, CAERN's water fee was R$1.39 per 10 cubic meters (equivalent to US$1.39 per 10 m^3).[59] In June 1995, the minimum water tariff (the rate charged to unmetered households) was R$3.81 per month (roughly equivalent to US$3.81 per month) and the minimum backyard condominial sewer charge (for unmetered households) was R$1.52 per month (roughly equivalent to US$1.52 per month). CAERN management staff reported that water fees were kept low for historical reasons, and that neither the water nor the sewer fees covered CAERN's true maintenance costs. Approximately 60 percent of CAERN's funds came from user fees paid by its customers in Natal—the remainder came from customers outside the capital city or from other sources.[60] Like COMPESA in Recife, CAERN also produced illustrated pamphlets to instruct residents on the proper use and maintenance of sewer systems. The information in CAERN's pamphlets was largely the same as that in COMPESA's.

This completes the introduction to the cities where condominial sewerage originated. Despite their differences, the cities of Natal and Recife are coastal capital cities of the Northeast region with a common history and culture of social exclusion indicated by high levels of poverty and inequitable access to infrastructure services. Both cities embraced condominial sewerage as a means to address inequity in the sanitation sector.

Growth of Condominial Sewerage during the Period of Innovation

During the years following the emergence of condominial sewers, very modest increases in water and sewer connections were made in the two leading capital cities that were implementing the technology in the Northeast (Recife and Natal).[61] Measured as the number of connections per 1,000 households, Recife added approximately 73 water connections, 12 condominial sewer connections, and –9 conventional sewer connections per 1,000 households during the 1987 to 1994 period (the rate of expansion of conventional sewer connections was negative because it was slower than the rate of population growth). In the 1990 to 1995 period,[62] Natal added water and sewer connections at the average rate of approximately 46 water connections, 12 condominial sewer connections, and –4 conventional sewer connections for every 1,000 households.

These rates of expansion (or reduction) in the number of connections relative to population indicate that Recife was adding water connections at a slightly faster rate than Natal, and that increases in water connections outpaced the respective population growth in each city during this period.[63] Natal had slightly more water connections per household than Recife at that time.[64] Conventional sewer expansion was insignificant in both cities during this period because the PLANASA era of federal investments in water and sanitation had come to an end. Neither city's rate of conventional sewer expansion exceeded the rate of population growth. In both cities, all of the growth in sewer connections was represented by condominial sewers. Although both cities had zero condominial sewer connections in 1980, by 1995 Natal's estimated condominial sewer coverage (79 connections per 1,000 households) was more than twice Recife's coverage (29 connections per 1,000 households).[65]

Recife and Natal increased their condominial sewer connections at nearly equal rates in the 1990s. However, by 1995 Natal had more condominial sewer connections per household than Recife because Natal had begun implementing condominial sewers in the early 1980s, approximately five years before Recife. The increases in sewer connections in Recife and Natal, although modest, consisted almost entirely of condominial sewer connections. Whereas few (if any) conventional sewer systems had been installed in favelas, poor, or low-income neighborhoods during the PLANASA era, the transition to condominial sewer technology allowed both Recife and Natal to begin extending sewerage to these previously unserved populations.

Closing Remarks for Chapter 3

This chapter introduced the sanitation conditions in the first two Brazilian cities to experiment with condominial sewerage. The Northeast capital cities of Natal and Recife offered contrasting contexts for observing the initial growth of condominial sewer projects. The urban geography of these two local settings was described, followed by a description of the range of sanitation situations faced by unserved residents, and an explanation of the governance structures in which services were delivered.

Notes

1. Pierre Bourdieu developed the important concept of *capital* and differentiated its forms, such as economic capital, social capital, cultural capital, and symbolic capital in Pierre Bourdieu, "The Forms of Capital," in *Handbook of Theory and Research for the Sociology of Education*, ed. J.G. Richardson (New York: Greenwood Press, 1986), 241–58.

2. Anthony Leeds, "Lower-Income Urban Settlement Types: Processes, Structures, Policies," in *The Residential Circumstances of the Urban Poor in Developing Countries*, United Nations Centre for Human Settlements (New York: Praeger Publishers, 1981); and Janice Perlman, *The Myth of Marginality: Urban Politics and Poverty in Rio de Janeiro* (Berkeley, CA: University of California Press, 1976).

3. Perlman, *The Myth of Marginality: Urban Politics and Poverty in Rio de Janeiro*, 168.

4. Perlman, *The Myth of Marginality: Urban Politics and Poverty in Rio de Janeiro.*

5. UFRJ-NCE Noticias, *Federal University of Rio de Janeiro Electronic Computer News*, 1993.

6. Perlman, *The Myth of Marginality: Urban Politics and Poverty in Rio de Janeiro*, 169.

7. Perlman, *The Myth of Marginality: Urban Politics and Poverty in Rio de Janeiro*, 240.

8. Helga Hoffman, "Poverty and Prosperity in Brazil: What Is Changing?," in *Social Change in Brazil, 1945--1985: The Incomplete Transition*, eds. Edmar L. Bacha and Herbert S. Klein (Albuquerque, NM: University of New Mexico Press, 1989).

9. World Bank, *World Development Report 1994: Infrastructure for Development* (Washington, DC: Oxford University Press, 1994).

10. Hoffman, "Poverty and Prosperity in Brazil: What Is Changing?"

11. Instituto Brasileiro de Geografia e Estatistica, *Brazil 2001* 2001, www.IBGE. gov.br/english/presidencia/noticias/12062003indic2002.shtm (19 Oct. 2005).

12. Virtual Brazil, "Minimum Wage in 2001," http://www.v-brazil.com/govern ment/executive-branch/lula/minimum-wage-2004.html (3 Oct. 2005).

13. Banco Central do Brasil, "Currency Exchange Rate for July 1, 2001," http://www5.bcb.gov.br/pec/taxas/ingl/ptaxnpesq.asp?id=quotations (3 Oct. 2005).

14. Hoffman, "Poverty and Prosperity in Brazil: What Is Changing?," 211.

15. United Nations, *Human Development Report* 2005, http://hdr.undp.org/reports /global/2005/pdf/hdr05_HDI.pdf (2 Oct. 2005); and Hoffman, "Poverty and Prosperity in Brazil: What Is Changing?," 199.

16. Timothy J. Power and J. Timmons Roberts, "A New Brazil? The Changing Sociodemographic Context of Brazilian Democracy," in *Democratic Brazil: Actors, Institutions, and Processes*, ed. Peter R. Kingstone and Timothy J. Power (Pittsburgh, PA: University of Pittsburgh Press, 2000), 248.

17. Hoffman, "Poverty and Prosperity in Brazil: What Is Changing?"

18. Instituto Brasileiro de Geografia e Estatistica, *PNAD (National Household Sample Survey Tables BR4.1, BR7.6a, and 7.1-15)*, 1999, http://www.ibge.gov.br/english /estatistica/populacao/trabalhorendimento/pnad99.shtm (19 Sept. 2003).

19. Martin T. Katzman, "Urbanization since 1945," in *Social Change in Brazil, 1945-1985: The Incomplete Transition*, eds. Edmar L. Bacha and Herbert S. Klein (Albuquerque, NM: University of New Mexico Press, 1989).

20. Gehan Sinnatamby, "Low Cost Sanitation Systems for Urban Peripheral Areas in Northeast Brazil," Ph.D. dissertation (Leeds, UK: The University of Leeds, 1983).

21. World Health Organization, "Global Water Supply and Sanitation Assessment 2000 Report" 2000, http://www.who.int/docstore/water_sanitation_health/Globassessment/Global1.htm#1.1 (29 Mar. 2004); and Pan American Health Organization, "Country Health Profile—Brazil" in *Health in the Americas* 1998, http://www.paho.org/english/sha/prflbra.htm (29 Mar. 2004).

22. Aurelio Menendez, "Access to Basic Infrastructure by the Urban Poor," *Economic Development Institute Policy Seminar Report 28* (Washington, DC: The World Bank, 1991).

23. Gabrielle Watson, consultant to the World Bank, personal communication with author, July 1993, Washington, DC.

24. Wikipedia, "Nordeste," http://en.wikipedia.org/wiki/Nordeste (2 Oct. 2005).

25. Sergio Sauer, "The World Bank and Land Reform in Brazil, Part II," *Land Research Action Network* 2003, http://www.landaction.org/display.php?article=134 (2 Oct. 2005), 1.

26. Sergio Sauer, "The World Bank and Land Reform in Brazil, Part II," *Land Research Action Network* 2003.

27. These calculations cover the period 1989 to 1999 using data from Instituto Brasileiro de Geografia e Estatistica, *Pesquisa Nacional por Amostra de Domicflios (National Household Sample Survey)* 1999, http://www.ibge.gov.br/english/estatistica/populacao/trabalhorendimento/pnad99/sintese/tab7_1_15.shtm (19 Sept. 2003).

28. World Bank, "Project Appraisal Document for the Recife Urban Upgrading Project," *Report No. 23331-BR* (Washington, DC: The World Bank, 2003).

29. Gustavo Valente, Brazilian citizen and civil engineer, personal communication with author, November 2003, Tracy, CA.

30. These calculations of the percentage of households in favelas cover the year 1999 for Recife and the year 2000 for Natal, using data from IBGE, 2003 (www.IBGE.gov.br).

31. The Inter-American Development Bank (IDB) categorizes small cities as having fewer than 100,000 people and medium cities as having between 100,000 to 500,000 people (Jaap De Vries, Micaela Schuster, Paul Procee, and Harry Mengers, "Environmental Management of Small and Medium Sized Cities in Latin America and the Caribbean," IDB Working Paper, Washington, DC, 2001, p. 1. Available at http://www.iadb.org/sds/ENV/publication/publication_195_2069_e.htm, accessed on October 2, 2005).

32. These calculations use data from the 2000 Brazilian Census (IBGE).

33. These calculations use data from COMPESA (1995) and CAERN (1995).

34. Informant 79, CAERN technical staff, interview by author, 24 April 1995, Natal, transcript; and Informant 76, CAERN social worker, interview by author, 10 May 1995, Natal, transcript.

35. Informant 31, consulting engineer, interview by author, 3 March 1995, Recife, transcript.

36. Information about condominial sewer implementation in Recife was obtained from interviews with engineers, participation staff, maintenance staff, managers, agency officials, elected officials, and engineering consultants. Key informants included Informants 1, 3, 4, 7, 9, 12, 16, 29, 30, 31, 59, 100, 101, 102, 103, 105, and 106; however many others also contributed. Other sources of information were also used, including project reports, maps, engineering drawings, memoranda, census records, newspaper clippings, interviews with residents, and other sources.

37. Information about condominial sewer implementation in Natal was obtained from interviews with engineers, participation staff, maintenance staff, managers, agency officials, elected officials, and engineering consultants. Key informants included Informants 75, 76, 77, 78, 83, 84, 87, 88, 89, 96, 98, 99, 120, 121, and 122, however many others also contributed. Other sources of information were also used, including project reports, maps, engineering drawings, memoranda, census records, newspaper clippings, interviews with residents, and other sources.

38. "Dreno" systems were installed by Recife's state water and sanitation agency to connect homes to an existing storm drain system. Some storm drain systems ultimately led to a low-level treatment system (such as a stabilization pond), but the majority of the storm drain systems discharged the sewage (or, in some cases, the solids-free wastewater) to a local water body.

39. Informant 59, a division chief for COMPESA, interview by author, March 20, 1995, Recife, transcript.

40. Informant 1, engineering consultant and former official, interview by author, 2 and 13 March 1995, Recife, transcript.

41. Informant 1, engineering consultant and former official, interview by author, 2 and 13 March 1995, Recife, transcript.

42. Informant 16, president of a Recife sewer agency, interview by author, March 16, 1995, Recife, transcript.

43. Informant 16, president of a Recife sewer agency, interview by author, 16 March 1995, Recife, transcript; and Informant 7, URB department chief, interview by author, 8 March 1995, Recife, transcript.

44. Interviews with residents of a Recife neighborhood, interviewed by Nance in 1994 and 1995, Recife, transcripts available.

45. Informant 76, CAERN social worker, interview with author, 30 May 1995, Natal, transcript.

46. OBRAS is an abbreviation for *Empresa de Obras Públicas*.

47. Informant 59, COMPESA division chief, interview by author, 20 March 1995, Recife, transcript.

48. Informant 12, COMPESA engineer, interview by author, 10 March 1995, Recife, transcript.

49. COMPESA, 1995.

50. COMPESA, 1995.

51. COMPESA billing records, 1995.

52. COMPESA, 1995.

53. The content and quality of CAERN's and COMPESA's sewer maintenance pamphlets were similar. See, for example, COMPESA (no date), *Sistema de Esgotamento Sanitário Manutencao do Sistema*, available at http://www.compesa.pe.gov.br.

54. Informant 83, CAERN, engineering director, interview with author, 4 July 1995, Natal, transcript.

55. Informant 75, CAERN senior civil engineer and sewer construction coordinator, interview with author, 24 May 1994, Natal, transcript.

56. Informant 75, CAERN senior civil engineer and sewer construction coordinator, interview with author, 24 May 1994, Natal, transcript.

57. Informant 75, CAERN senior civil engineer and sewer construction coordinator, interview with author, 25 May 1995, Natal, transcript.

58. CAERN sewer billing records, 1995.

59. Informant 98, CAERN director president of a Natal sewer agency, interview with author, 6 June 1995, Natal, transcript.

60. Informant 76, CAERN social worker, interview with author, 11 April 1995, Natal, transcript; and Informant 88, CAERN condominial sewer technician, interview with author, 11 May 1995, Natal, transcript.

61. Other Brazilian cities outside the Northeast, such as the city of Sao Paulo, had far greater resources and made far greater increases in water and sanitation services, as detailed by Watson, 1992.

62. These time periods reflect the first year that computerized records were kept in Recife (1987) and Natal (1990), and the year for which data on water connections were available during my fieldwork in Recife (1994/1995) and Natal (1995).

63. The Recife and Natal time periods are slightly different because connection data for Natal were not available prior to 1990.

64. Possible explanations for this are that Natal could have exhibited higher rates of water system expansion in previous years, or that Recife could have counted more of its unconnected households (i.e., poor households) than Natal. On the second possible explanation, it is instructive to know that Recife had more favelas within its boundaries than Natal, and that Recife had granted land title to many of its favelas, while Natal had not. Consequently, the "unofficial" favelas in Natal may not have been counted as unconnected households. It is also instructive to know that Natal's population growth during that time (14 percent) exceeded Recife's population growth (9 percent).

65. These estimates of the expansion of water and sewer connections per thousand households in Recife and Natal were calculated using data on the number of service connections from COMPESA (1994) and CAERN (1995); city household data from IBGE-Malha (1997); and city population data from Populstat (2003).

Chapter 4
Participation and Alignment in the City of Natal

Natal was the first city to innovate with condominial sewers. In the 1980s and 1990s, progressive elected officials and activist engineers created and experimented with a new sanitation approach in an attempt to serve low-income residents. What conditions allowed them to succeed and what challenges did they have to overcome? Part of the answer lies in whether or not interests were aligned among key decision-making officials. The alignment of interests between elected officials and implementing organizations had a significant effect on project outcome during the 1980s and early 1990s.

While political parties changed at every election, for most of the 1980s each state and local administration gave the state water and sanitation agency (*Companhia de Águas e Esgotos do Rio Grande do Norte*, or CAERN) a degree of autonomy in implementing condominial sewers in Natal. From 1980 through 1990, there was consistent support for condominial sewers by elected officials and by CAERN engineers. This unusual period of stability is a notable characteristic of Natal's implementation success in the 1980s. In the 1990s, however, these alignments began to shift. One visible shift was the lack of enthusiastic support for condominial sewers from a newly elected governor in 1991 and from his appointed director of CAERN, as reported by condominial sewer practitioners who were actively involved in project implementation during the period. Precipitating this weakening of support was the expiration of CAERN's contract with the City of Natal in 1992, and the national decentralization of funding from state governments to municipal governments that occurred in the early 1990s. The overall result was a four-year period (1991–1994) in which no condominial sewers were implemented in Natal. A second indication of shifting alignments was the election of a new mayor in 1994 who strongly promoted municipal control and quasi-privatization of Natal's sewer system. By this time, the City Urbanization Agency (*Empresa da Urbanização do Natal*, or URBANA) was competing with CAERN for project funds and for decision-making authority over sewer development in Natal. This signaled the end of Natal's initial period of condominial sewer innovation.

This chapter introduces the concept "alignment of interests" to express a key result of Natal's condominial sewer experience from 1980 to 1995. I present a timeline of events that characterize the evolution of alignments during the period, I offer measures of condominial sewer performance during the period, and I introduce possible partial explanations of the relationship between the alignment of interests and project performance. I bring the concept "alignment of interests" (or "alignments") into the discussion as convenient shorthand to refer to a particular set of actions and as a way to focus the analysis and the narrative.

Alignment of Interests: A Critical Concept

One observation that emerges from Natal's innovation period is that the existence of condominial sewer projects was linked to how interests were aligned between elected officials and the state water and sanitation company. As an empirical concept, "alignment of interests" attempts to capture one of the most critical aspects of implementation with respect to overall performance. One can think of alignment of interests as an invisible aspect of condominial sewer performance; an aspect that links the political and the material together. My observations of Natal's innovation period yielded four types of alignments that were important to condominial sewer outcomes: 1) elected officials and implementing organizations had varying interests in being responsive to or representative of popular needs; 2) elected officials and implementing agencies had varying interests in their desire to serve as spokespersons for condominial sewer technology as an alternative to conventional sewer technology; 3) elected officials in one political regime had varying interests in expressing a continuity of support for sanitation projects introduced by the previous regime; and 4) city and state implementing agencies had varying interests in coordinating with each other on sanitation projects.

In the first type of alignment I hypothesize that the existence of condominial sewers was enhanced when elected officials and implementing organizations were aligned in being responsive to the needs of the poor and middle class. Historical trends in Brazil are consistent with this hypothesis. Before democratization, local level units of state organs that implemented sewer projects were supportive of elites and were either neglectful or repressive toward the needs of the poor and the middle class.[1] This changed somewhat with the introduction of democratization in Brazil in the early 1980s. Democratization was accompanied by a wave of political interest in meeting the needs of the masses, especially with regard to urban services. Through fiscal decentralization, municipalities were granted direct access to infrastructure funds and, as a result, they acquired more autonomy. Samuels (2000) argues that municipal, state, and even federal politicians became particularly interested in serving urban areas as a result of the fiscal decentralization policies of the 1988 Brazilian Constitution.[2] The status and prestige of the position of mayor increased significantly from this point forward, demonstrated by the increasing number of state and federal level politicians who sought the position of mayor after the late 1980s and through the 1990s. Newly-elected mayors and governors who were responsive to popular needs often appointed like-minded individuals to run condominial sewer implementing organizations and to develop projects that would meet popular needs. Policy innovations, such as condominial sewers and the approach of involving beneficiaries in project implementation activities, flourished in the new political environment created by fiscal decentralization. Natal's innovation with condominial sewers as a specific means to serve poor residents will be explored later in the chapter as a prime example of the first alignment of interests.

In the second type of alignment I hypothesize that the emergence and presence of condominial sewers was linked to the emergence and presence of people willing to speak for condominial sewer technology. During Natal's innovation period condominial sewers were an emerging technology in Brazil, but this new technology was not broadly supported by the traditional representatives of water and sewerage systems. Indeed, some water and sanitation organizations and some elected officials actively opposed condominial sewer technology. Some condominial sewer projects were implemented by organizations and officials that accepted and embraced the technology; these organizations typically hired social scientists to implement the participation aspects of project implementation, and these organizations developed cadres of condominial sewer specialists within their organizations. Other condominial sewer projects were implemented by organizations and officials that did not believe in the technology or in participation. Later in the chapter Natal's experience during the 1980s and 1990s is used to illustrate both the presence and absence of condominial sewer spokespersons and the corresponding performance effects that occurred as this alignment of interests shifted.

In the third type of alignment I hypothesize that continuity from one political regime to the next was associated with condominial sewer performance; that is, projects could not maintain their existence or degree of performance over time without continuity. I observed that some condominial sewer projects were begun and completed within a single political regime, while other projects lost political support and funding because of a change in regime at some point during project implementation. Scholars have noted the chaotic nature of Brazilian politics and the persistence, even after the democratic opening in the 1980s, of an individualist political culture in which elected officials serve their own interests.[3] Within this individualistic political culture, as new leaders were elected and new regimes were installed, little or no value was given to maintaining continuity in the policies, projects, or employees of the previous regime. Even "basic needs" projects such as water and sanitation were politicized to a high degree, meaning that individual condominial sewer projects were tightly linked to their representatives. Projects were offered as patronage by elected officials who were linked to specific neighborhoods or population segments. Moreover, when a new official was elected, he or she frequently abandoned the projects initiated by the previous official because those projects represented the patronage of that official. This practice was not exclusive to one political party; leftist, centrist, and rightist politicians all carried out the custom. During a regime change, it was difficult for individual projects to keep their old representatives or attract new representatives. Later in the chapter we see the effects of continuity and discontinuity on project performance by observing how the alignment of interests changed during Natal's innovation period.

In the fourth type of alignment I hypothesize that variations in the degree of collaboration among city and state organizations corresponded with variations in condominial sewer performance. For some projects, the implementing organizations interacted with each other in a coordinated manner to implement condominial sewer projects; while other projects experienced lack of coordination, competition, or even alienation among implementing organizations. Scholars have noted the lack of vertical (state-city) and horizontal (city-city or state-state) coordination between Brazil's governmental organizations since democratization and the concurrent wave of decentralization.[4] Since the 1980s, Brazilian organizations at the same level of government and organizations at different levels of government typically have had increased difficulty working together.[5] Further in the chapter we will see periods of coordinated implementation of condominial sewers followed by increasing destabilization of the coalition of condominial sewer organizations and the cumulative performance effects of this shifting alignment of interests.

The following sections describe key events of Natal's innovation period. The period is discussed in three parts on the basis of the four alignments just described. These three sections are summarized in Table 4-1.

A Decade of Durable Alignments: 1980–1990

The decade of the 1980s was, by all accounts, the most successful period of implementation the City of Natal had experienced. The period 1980–1990 had been deemed the "International Water and Sanitation Decade" by the World Bank. During the "Decade," significant global resources were made available for the purpose of increasing access to water and sanitation services through appropriate designs and participatory approaches. In Brazil, this policy objective first took shape in the Northeast region of the country. During the first seven years of the decade (1980–1986), Josemar Azevedo served as President of the CAERN Directorate. President Josemar (known popularly by his first name) was supported by Lúcio Flávio as Directorate Engineer and Valmir Rocha as Directorate Administrator. These were the top water and sanitation officials of the state, and they were fortunate to have a long time period in which to innovate—a rarity in Brazil.

Table 4-1. Timeline of events related to the condominial sewer innovation period in Natal from 1980 to 1995.

Year	Events
	Durable Alignments
1980	The state water and sanitation agency, CAERN, received funds for the implementation of the first condominial sewer system in Natal, Rio Grande do Norte.
1982	CAERN President Josemar Azevedo provided enthusiastic and consistent support of condominial sewer technology. The first condominial sewers in Natal were completed in the neighborhoods of Rocas and Santos Reis. CAERN received additional funds for more condominial sewers throughout the state.
1983	CAERN presented its condominial sewer experience in an engineering conference in Santa Catarina, Brazil. A wave of interest in condominial sewer technology spread through Brazil's water and sanitation industry.
1987	Support for condominial sewer projects continued, but access to new project funding started to shrink following 1986 changes in federal finance rules. CAERN began charging sewer tariffs to condominial sewer beneficiaries, computerized its records, and focused on maintaining existing projects instead of implementing new projects.
1988	Brazil's first Constitution was ratified, empowering cities to receive direct financing for water and sewer infrastructure. Implementation of this change did not occur in Natal until the early 1990s.
	Weakening Alignments
1991	CAERN President Walter Gomez implemented condominial sewers in Basin I using funds leftover from the previous administration. The lack of enthusiastic support and the lack of new funding led to the paralysis of condominial sewer implementation.
1992	CAERN's twenty-year water and sanitation service contract with the City of Natal expired.
1994	Conflict began between CAERN and the City of Natal. Mayor Aldo Tinoco Filho promoted the quasi-privatization of a new treatment plant and sewer system in Natal and the development of a water and sanitation division within City government. CAERN and the City of Natal each received new project funds and began implementing condominial sewer projects simultaneously.
	Destabilizing Alignments
1995	CAERN President Luiz Jorge Coelho Leal used the funding received at the end of the previous administration to implement the Basin I project. CAERN also received funding to complete the Basin D project. CAERN underwent a major re-organization in which the agency was decentralized.

Sources: CAERN staff members, interviews by author, 1995, Natal, transcripts; and http://www.natal.br.gov.

After the initial pilot projects in Rocas, Santos Reis, and several interior towns in the early 1980s, CAERN installed thousands of condominial sewer connections in Natal over the next ten years. These connections were located in five sewer basins throughout the city (i.e., Basins A, C, D, E, and K). Much of the financing for these projects came from the World Bank's Medium-Size Cities Program and the 1984–1988 State Program (*Programa do Estado*).[6]

Josemar Azevedo served an unprecedented two consecutive terms as President of the CAERN Directorate during this time—unprecedented because his terms overlapped with three different governors who each represented different political parties. Josemar's two terms covered eight of the eleven years that comprised the period of durable alignments (1980–1987). For the first two years of Josemar's term (1980–1981), the governor had been appointed by the military regime. For the next four years of Josemar's presidency (1982–1985), José Agripino Maia of the rightist Party of the Liberal Front (PFL) (who was now elected rather than appointed) served as governor (1982–1985). For the final two years of Josemar's presidency (1986–1987), Geraldo José da Câmara Ferreira de Melo of the centrist Party of the Brazilian Democratic Movement (PMDB) served as governor.

During the first decade of condominial sewerage, CAERN's Directorate, led by Azevedo, played a direct role in condominial sewer development, and the Governor's office played a lesser role. CAERN employees reported that none of the governors during the 1980–1990 period expressed much interest in condominial sewers, per se. Consequently the CAERN Directorate, which was appointed by the governor, was able to act quasi-autonomously with regard to condominial sewer development. The municipal government of Natal also had little or no influence on CAERN with regard to condominial sewers during this initial period. CAERN's relative autonomy was enhanced by its direct access to federal funds during the first seven years of the period of durable alignments (1980–1986). The Directorate used its access to the governor as necessary to facilitate their search for project funds.

During this period CAERN had the time, resources, and autonomy to experiment with and develop a proven approach for implementing condominial sewers. CAERN's participation program included the following:

- Mobilizing residents to encourage widespread support for the project;
- Mobilizing residents to educate them about the benefits of sanitary sewers;
- Involving residents in project decisions;
- Obtaining contributions from residents in project construction;
- Obtaining commitments from residents to contribute to project maintenance.

CAERN staff members cited the lack of user education as a primary reason for misuse of condominial sewer systems by users.[7] Several CAERN employees were unsatisfied with the way CAERN's participation program was used to educate beneficiaries about sewer system maintenance.[8] They felt that one block meeting or house visit was not enough to be effective in fully educating beneficiaries about their condominial sewer; and that ongoing education about how to perform maintenance was more likely to promote proper use and maintenance of the system.[9]

The content of CAERN's participation program in Natal varied slightly from project to project. But few, if any, condominial sewer projects were implemented without participation.[10] Resident involvement (i.e., the percentage of residents who participated) in CAERN's participation program varied by block for every project. CAERN's level of investment in its participation program also varied from project to project.[11] According to practitioners in Natal, the levels of resident involvement actually experienced in condominial sewer projects were typically 30 percent of the neighborhood population (with typical highs of 40–50 percent); however, levels as high as 100 percent involvement, although very rare, were also reported.[12] Attendance rates above 50 percent were considered good.[13] CAERN participation staff members did a number of things to facilitate resident involvement and the development of user groups (called *condomínios or pactos condominios*), which CAERN considered important for project success. CAERN employees contacted residents directly, administered questionnaires, distributed meeting invitations, posted fliers, held meetings, and had informal conversations with residents.

Given the low levels of education and literacy of residents in most low-income and poor neighborhoods, written invitations to project meetings were not always effective. CAERN used speaker cars (*carros de som*) to invite residents to project meetings and found this to be very effective. A person sitting inside the speaker car made announcements into a microphone that transmitted their voice through giant speakers mounted on the roof of the car. The car was driven through the neighborhood so that as many residents as possible would hear the announcement.

Typically 30 percent of residents on a given block attended participation meetings held by CAERN prior to the construction of a condominial sewer project. The objectives of these meetings were to educate residents about sanitation, inform them about the condominial sewer system, distribute educational pamphlets, motivate the formation of a user group, and convince as many residents as possible to accept a sewer connection, authorize construction, and agree to perform maintenance. CAERN's participation program meetings included the experimental use of theater groups (*teatros*). At first, the theater groups were included in block-by-block project meetings. Amateur actors performed skits to educate residents on the benefits and operation of the condominial sewer system. But because only fifteen to twenty residents were typically present for each block meeting, it was decided that this was not a big enough audience to justify the time and energy involved in preparing and performing the skits multiple times. The theater groups were then moved to local schools to educate students about sewers and sanitation.

For the 70 percent of residents that did not attend a typical project meeting, CAERN's student interns and vocational school graduates went house-to-house to explain the project and to obtain the signatures of residents who were interested in hooking up. Typically, the end of CAERN's participation program coincided with the end of project construction. As a result, only the implementation staff (not the operations and maintenance staff) was involved in the participation program. Despite the fact that the participation program included education about how to perform maintenance, and that user maintenance was a goal of the participation program, maintenance staff was not involved in the participation program.

In 1987, Luiz Roberto was appointed President of the CAERN Directorate by Governor Geraldo Melo. João Felipe Medeiros was appointed Directorate Engineer, and Roger Mariz was appointed Directorate Administrator. This Directorate served until 1990, the end of the period of durable alignments. The timing of President Roberto's administration coincided with a change in federal funding arrangements and an increased difficulty in acquiring funding. In 1986, the National Housing Bank (*Banco Nacional da Habitação,* or BNH) had been disbanded and replaced by the Federal Bank of Brazil (*Caixa Econômica Federal,* or CEF); and funding from PLANASA ended in 1987. In 1988, Brazil's new Constitution was ratified, which decentralized federal financing of the sanitation sector and transferred some responsibilities to municipalities.[14] Because new project funding was becoming more difficult to obtain, President Roberto was only able to continue implementing condominial sewers using resources left over from the previous administration of President Azevedo. Roberto did continue to support the innovation and made attempts to institutionalize it. He increased the agency's focus on maintenance activities and integrated the group of specialized condominial sewer engineers into the regular staff of CAERN. The condominial sewer specialists were integrated across the three major divisions of the agency (i.e., the Projects, Construction, and Operations Divisions).

During the first decade, condominial sewers in Natal were installed in sewer basin A (a large pilot project in the Rocas and Santos Reis neighborhoods), in sewer basin C (small projects in the Tirol and Lagoa Seca neighborhoods), in sewer basin K (a small project in the Felipe Camarão neighborhood), and in sewer basins D and E (large projects in the Quintas, Nordeste, Alecrim, Bom Pastor, and Dix-Sept Rosado neighborhoods). Most of the condominial sewer funding received by CAERN in this period came with the condition that it be applied only in low-income or poor areas. With a few exceptions, all of the neighborhoods listed above were low-income or poor; however, none were favelas.

Weakening Alignments: 1991–1994

The period from 1991 through 1994 brought a complete interruption in condominial sewer development in Natal resulting from CAERN's reduced ability to obtain funds for new projects and from a breakdown in the alignment of interests supporting the new approach. In 1991, Walter Gomez was appointed president of the CAERN Directorate by Governor José Agripino Maia, who had just been elected to his second (non-consecutive) term under the rightist PFL party (recall that Agripino had been governor during the first half of the previous decade). Francisco Pancracio Madruga was appointed Directorate Engineer, and Rui Barbosa was appointed Directorate Administrator.

Despite the innovations of the previous decade, President Gomez substituted key condominial sewer employees within CAERN with new employees who did not understand or support the original condominial sewer approach. Gomez did not initially seek new condominial sewer project funding; rather he used funds that were leftover from the previous administration. Because of this, some employees believed that this Directorate was not as supportive of condominial sewer technology as previous Directorates. Other employees reported that the Directorate wanted to seek new funds, but was limited by the new financing rules and a more difficult implementing environment.

In October 1992, CAERN's twenty-year contract with Natal expired. The City of Natal had not developed the know-how, the staff, or the equipment to manage its water and sanitation infrastructure alone. Despite this, the City did not immediately renew their contract with CAERN as most interior cities had done. During this "no contract" period, CAERN continued to provide water and sanitation services on an interim basis while City officials decided what to do about the contract. Despite CAERN's past efforts and modest progress in developing water and sanitation services in Natal, the agency's entire role in Natal was now being questioned due to higher expectations for progress and system expansion.

Notwithstanding the diminished funding for new projects, existing funding for projects already being implemented was abruptly halted by the CAERN Directorate. One project in Natal was paralyzed after only 77 percent of the condominial sewers (54 of 70 blocks) and 16 percent of the house connections (900 of 5,500 connections) were completed. Beneficiaries who lived on the completed blocks took the initiative to finish constructing their house connections during the project down time. One advantage of the project stoppage was that it allowed time for house connection construction to catch up to the level of construction progress already achieved in the rest of project.[15]

The original specialized condominial sewer staff members maintained their employment in CAERN through the various phases of support in the 1980s and non-support in the 1990s. Individuals took assignments in different departments of CAERN, and the individuals could be reconvened as a group whenever implementation of condominial sewer projects started up again. CAERN staff members who had been part of the original specialized group that implemented condominial sewers during the first decade of innovation were particularly frustrated with this period of weakening alignments.[16] During times of funding paralysis, the specialized condominial professionals within CAERN prepared and submitted funding proposals and put together engineering plans for the extension of condominial sewers into new basins. Knowing that the implementing environment eventually would become favorable again, they wanted to be ready to implement as many new projects as possible during the next period of support. Finished proposals and plans were piled up on the shelf, waiting for the next shift in alliances that would either support or prevent the expansion of condominial sewerage.

It did take CAERN some time to figure out how to access new sources of funding in the new environment. Toward the end of his term (in 1994), Gomez finally received condominial sewer funding from the German Development Bank for sewer basin I in Natal. There would be little time for his administration to implement the project, however.

Destabilizing Alignments: Post-1995

In 1995, Luiz Jorge Coelho Leal was appointed President of the CAERN Directorate by the newly elected Governor Garibaldi Alves Filho of the centrist PMDB party. Celso Veiga was appointed Directorate Engineer and Ismael Wanderly was appointed Directorate Administrator. Some condominial sewer staff members expected a continuation of project paralysis during the President Jorge administration. Unexpectedly, President Jorge did not redirect the project funding for sewer basin I that had been received at the end of the previous administration, thereby showing indirect support for continued expansion of condominial sewers in Natal. At the beginning of President Jorge's term, CAERN received additional funds from the Inter-American Development Bank (IDB) in 1994 (US$9 million from the PROSEGE Program), and was able to restart implementation of the condominial sewer projects that had been abruptly stopped. Despite this, some CAERN employees characterized this period as "a continuation of the indifference toward condominial sewer technology that had begun in the 1990–1994 period, because of the lack of effort and commitment to seek new funds."[17] In the words of one CAERN staff member:[18]

> In the old days [of the 1970s and 1980s], the CAERN Directorate would go to Brasilia [the federal capital] in search of project money, until about four years ago [in 1990] when it changed. Now the mayors, deputies, and senators go to Brasilia in search of money and they hire CAERN to do the project and the maintenance. It was better when CAERN sought funds. Today CAERN's continuing expenses are a problem, since it only gets funds on a project basis. CAERN gets less money with the new decentralized system.

Another complaint of some CAERN employees was that as the number of condominial sewer connections in Natal grew, there was no additional funding to augment the operations and maintenance department. They made this complaint because most international lenders and funding sources only provided new project money, not money to maintain existing projects. Maintenance funds were supposed to be provided by the home country government and from user fees. The combination of CAERN's dwindling access to federal funding and its financially unsustainable sewer fee structure were the reasons behind this complaint.

CAERN revised its participation approach further for the condominial sewer projects implemented after 1995. In the original approach applied in the early 1980s, CAERN provided the materials and constructed the house connections for residents. In its revised approach of the late 1980s, CAERN provided the house connection materials, and residents constructed or contracted the construction of their house connections. Thousands of connections had been installed in this manner, with plumbing contractors being paid directly by the residents. The consequence of this change was that newly constructed projects could no longer be immediately transferred to CAERN's maintenance division because of the need to wait for the majority of residents to construct their house connections.[19] By 1995, CAERN decided to stop providing house connection materials. Residents were now expected to install their own condominial sewer connections without any financial assistance from CAERN. The residents had to buy their own materials and install the connections themselves or hire a contractor. CAERN reasoned that residents would do this if they were genuinely interested in having a sewer. Participation by residents therefore increased over time, not as a result of project outcomes but in response to changes in the implementing environment.

These changes in CAERN's program indicate that residents now were expected to contribute more than they had in previous years. Interestingly, however, one staff member characterized the changes in CAERN's expectations of what beneficiaries should do as a reduction in participation rather than an increase.[20] This staff member said that participation in the 1980–1990 period—such as in the Rocas and Santos Reis projects—was "better" than in 1995 because CAERN made more of an investment in its participation program, and because residents were more interested in the condominial sewer systems. This employee argued that as projects got bigger over the years, the pace of construction increased and it was no longer possible to perform all of the participation program activities that had previously been performed with the same number of employees. In other words, CAERN's participation program became relatively smaller over time.

CAERN's post-1995 implementation of condominial sewers evolved in other ways as well. Design was simplified by the use of standard sizes and off-the-shelf parts instead of custom-sized systems that required detailed calculations and non-standard parts. Financial technicians were now included in participation meetings to answer questions and to assist residents with house connection finance issues. CAERN also started documenting its participation process in written reports for the first time, beginning with the post-1995 projects in sewer basins I and D.[21]

Reflecting on the overall problems they faced, CAERN engineering employees noted that the two areas most needing improvement were system performance and lack of maintenance. One senior CAERN staff member reported that "there is a contract between CAERN and residents for the residents to do their own operation and maintenance, but CAERN ends up doing it."[22] He continued to say, "only functioning [of condominial sewers] had not improved." Other employees made similar statements. Less frequently mentioned was the problem of maintaining the *condominios*, or resident user groups.

Despite the innovation and sustained efforts of CAERN, by 1995 only about 20 percent of Natal's residents had access to sewer systems. This striking statistic overshadowed CAERN's years of commitment to developing and disseminating condominial sewer technology, implementing condominial sewer projects, and perfecting its participation program. Despite its success in using participation to implement projects in low-, middle-, and high-income areas, CAERN had not been able to expand this success over time, partly because of changes in federal funding arrangements, increasing expectations, and increasing population. In the words of one high-level City official, the achievement of only 20 percent sewer coverage over twenty years was an indication of CAERN's ineffectiveness.[23]

This sense of failure dovetailed with an increased global interest in the privatization of state enterprises, and consequently resulted in a period of transition and destabilization during which attempts were made to redirect CAERN's role and privatize certain aspects of sanitation service. In 1995, the Mayor of Natal and the President of Natal's Urbanization Agency (*Empresa de Urbanização do Natal*, or URBANA) began negotiating with a private firm. The negotiations centered around a potential thirty-year contract for the design, construction, operation, and maintenance of a new sewage treatment plant and sewer system extension. CAERN's proposed role would be to administer the billing of new customers. This represented a very significant reduction in responsibility compared to what CAERN had done in the past and an increase in the City's direct role.

Historically, Natal's municipal government had not been directly involved in water and sanitation functions, and had only expressed a passive interest in the subject.[24] The City and CAERN had not worked closely together in the past, because the City had relied entirely on CAERN to provide water and sanitation services. But in 1994 a former CAERN civil engineer, Aldo Tinoco Filho, was elected Mayor of Natal under the center left Party of Brazilian Social Democracy (PSDB). With the election of an engineer-mayor who had experience implementing condominial sewers, Natal's City government became more interested in developing the capacity to independently manage its water and sanitation sector. Collectively, the City's newfound interest in taking more responsibility for local water and sanitation, the federal government's empowerment of cities through the decentralization of project funding arrangements, the global privatization movement of the 1990s (promoted by the World Bank), and the growing dissatisfaction with CAERN's lack of progress combined to create an atmosphere of conflict between the City and CAERN. Both CAERN and URBANA could now compete independently for funds from the federal government (e.g., from the *Banco Nacional Desenvolvimento Social*, or National Bank of Social Development) or from international lending agencies (e.g., the World Bank).

City and CAERN employees now openly criticized the agency, describing CAERN as a "paternalistic bureaucracy." To quote one official, "CAERN is the mother and the father and wants to do everything for the people." CAERN's practice of performing maintenance on condominial sewers was noted as evidence of its paternalistic culture. Opponents viewed CAERN's maintenance decisions as a major error in policy implementation, because condominial sewer beneficiaries had signed contracts (called *Adhesão de Serviço* or *Cartas de Adhesão*) obligating them to do their own maintenance, although these contracts were not legally binding. In 1995, a senior CAERN official reported that "relations between CAERN and the City are the worse they've ever been now that Aldo is Mayor."[25]

During this period of destabilization, URBANA applied for and received US$3 million from IDB's PROSEGE Program to implement the first City-led condominial sewer project. Two units within the City government were assigned to the project: URBANA and the Municipal Public Works Division (*Superintendência Municipal de Obras e Viação*, or SUMOV). The City government also decentralized itself and installed offices in the four administrative regions of the city to increase its local community presence. URBANA implemented the City's first condominial sewer project at the same time CAERN was using its own PROSEGE funds to complete unfinished condominial sewer projects from the 1980s. URBANA reported that it was able to construct its entire project (three thousand connections for fifteen thousand residents) for only US$840,000, which was less than one-third of the estimated cost.[26] URBANA's cost per sewer connection (or "unit" cost) was much lower than CAERN's unit cost, and the City used this fact as evidence that it could utilize sanitation funds more efficiently than CAERN. The mayor, the governor, and the president of URBANA all supported the idea of creating a municipal water and sewer agency (*Companhia Municipal de Saneamento*) to implement water, sewer, solid waste, and drainage infrastructure services in Natal. CAERN publicly supported the proposal even though the agency did not agree with Natal's desire to privatize some components of its sanitation infrastructure.

During this period of destabilization, CAERN implemented a new condominial project in sewer basin I and continued implementation of an existing condominial sewer project in sewer basin D. Also, other international lending organizations (beyond the World Bank) became involved in condominial sewer project financing, including the Bank of Germany and the Inter-American Development Bank.

Alignment and Participation as Elements of Performance

This chapter has covered condominial sewer implementation in the City of Natal from 1980 to 1995. The discussion highlighted two central themes relevant to condominial sewerage. First, the decade of the 1980s was an important period of innovation in Natal. There was relative stability in the alignment of interests supporting condominial sewers 1980 to 1990; but after 1990 the implementing environment disintegrated as indicated by weakening and destabilizing alignment of interests in condominial sewers. Second, there was overall coherence in how condominial sewers were implemented, with a single approach being perfected and revised over time by a single agency using a centralized approach. Natal's practitioners stressed the importance of the participatory process,[27] and consistently practiced a participation program in which beneficiaries were involved in all aspects of project implementation, including mobilization of residents, project decision-making, project construction, and project maintenance. This participation program evolved and changed during the period, but CAERN's commitment to having a participation program was unwavering. CAERN was able to learn by trial and error how to deliver sanitation services to previously unserved neighborhoods; however, CAERN's overall performance was contested on the basis of low connection rates.

Expansion in the number of sewer connections during Natal's innovation period was difficult to obtain for two reasons. First, the planned number of connections was different than the number of connections actually built, so project planning documents, engineering reports, and blueprints often overstated the actual number of connections. Second, all households in Natal's sewered areas were charged a monthly sewer fee whether they were connected or not. CAERN's reason for doing this was that sewers were considered a public good. Because everyone in a project area received the benefits of the sewer, everyone was expected to contribute to its cost. As a result of this billing approach, billing records may have further overstated the number of connections. Nevertheless, billing records were still one of the best sources of information for tracking growth in the total number of connections because the records were continually updated. The first condominial sewers in Natal were completed in 1982. Sewer tariffs were not charged until 1986–1987, around the same time that CAERN computerized its records. Consequently, CAERN's billing records and sewer connection information prior to 1986 did not include any information about condominial sewers, since these early connections were not yet being charged. In 1995, CAERN billing records showed 17,282 conventional sewer units billed, 12,752 condominial sewer units billed, and 148,519 water units billed.

CAERN employees estimated that approximately 20–25 percent of Natal's population was sewered by 1995 (conventional and condominial sewers), and that about 90 percent of the condominial sewer connections were for low-income and poor residents. Middle-income and high-income beneficiaries made up the remaining 10 percent of condominial sewer beneficiaries. On the basis of census data, only 19 percent of the 0.7 million people in Natal had access to sewers (not including septic tanks) and 95 percent had access to water in 1994.

Despite the relatively low sewer-access rate across the city, by 1995 Natal had a good overall record of performance for the projects that were installed. The majority of condominial sewer projects that were initiated in the 1980–1990 period were either completed or in the process of being completed. Most of these projects functioned adequately (as of 1995), and most projects had a suitable destination for the collected sewage[28] (although the sewage treatment plant was barely maintained). Project representatives I interviewed characterized Natal's overall performance as "good" when choosing among the categories "bad," "fair," "good," "very good," and "excellent."[29] This characterization is supported by a separate World Bank-commissioned condominial sewer survey,[30] in which Natal's overall project performance was characterized as "good" on an excellent/good/bad scale compared to six other Brazilian cities.

Closing Remarks for Chapter 4

This chapter revealed how multiple factors and forces came together in the City of Natal to produce the first condominial sewer projects. The story involved activist engineers who were willing to champion a new technology and a participatory approach. Both of these innovations directly challenged the status quo and required the engineers to act strategically so they would be allowed the freedom to experiment. The chapter also revealed Natal's response to the decentralizing milieu it found itself in as the nation was establishing a democracy. Natal was unusual because of its initial resistance to decentralization in the water and sanitation sector. The chapter showed how success in this urban setting required the creation and maintenance of a coalition of support for each individual project.

The specific conditions of condominial sewer emergence in Natal that were presented in this chapter revealed competing narratives among those who speak for sanitation technology. Opponents of condominial sewer technology argued for its failure on the basis of the low connection rate that was achieved. Proponents of the technology emphasized the innovative learning that took place during the period of innovation, resulting in perceptions of success measured in terms of project quality, bottom-up participation, and top-down support for bringing sewers to previously unserved areas of the city. Without essentializing the 1980-1995 period, one leaves this chapter with a sense that project performance was good initially and then declined, and that alignments shifted from stable to weak and then finally destabilized. We saw how four types of alignments played out over Natal's innovation period, which raises interesting questions. Did alignment of interests "cause" condominial sewers to perform, or did performance "cause" interests to align? Or did the relationship between the two take place within a larger network of actors serving to link development discourse to development outcomes in new and different ways? These questions arise yet cannot be answered at this point in the book. Nevertheless, knowing the status of the four alignments in a particular time and place will be an important element of the answer. As I continue to interrogate the implications of condominial sewerage as an inclusive development practice, I will revisit both "performance" and "alignments" in ways that bring more narratives to bear on these questions.

Notes

1. Mainwaring, 1989, 178.
2. Samuels, 2000, 92.
3. Skidmore, 1989; Mainwaring, 1989; Samuels, 2000, 97; and Mainwaring, 1999.
4. Samuels, 2000, 95.
5. Samuels, 2000.
6. Informant 1, engineering consultant, former municipal official, former state official, interview with author, March 1995, Recife, transcript; and Informant 75, CAERN senior civil engineer and sewer construction coordinator, interview with author, 24 May 1995, Natal, transcript.
7. Informant 76, CAERN social worker, interview with author, 11 April 1995, Natal, transcript.
8. Informant 76, CAERN social worker, interviews with author, 11 April 1995 and 30 May 1995, Natal, transcripts; Informant 120, URBANA civil engineer, interview with author, 31 May 1995, Natal, transcript; and Informant 78, CAERN sewer design division chief, interview with author, 24 May 1995, Natal, transcript.
9. Informant 76, CAERN social worker, interview with author, 11 April 1995, Natal, transcript; and Informant 120, URBANA civil engineer, interview with author, 31 May 1995, Natal, transcript.
10. Informant 75, CAERN senior civil engineer and sewer construction coordinator, interview with author, 17 April 1995, Natal, transcript.
11. Informant 85, CAERN participation staff member, interview with author, 11 May 1995, Natal, transcript.
12. Informant 75, CAERN senior civil engineer and sewer construction coordinator, interviews with author, 23 May 1995 and 24 May 1995, Natal, transcript; Informant 120, URBANA civil engineer, interview with author, 31 May 1995, Natal, transcript; interview with Informant 75, CAERN senior civil engineer and sewer construction coordinator, 24 May 1994, Natal.
13. Informant 75, CAERN senior civil engineer and sewer construction coordinator, interview with author, 23 May 1995, Natal, transcript.
14. Samuels, 2000, 82–83, 93.
15. Informant 120, URBANA civil engineer, interview with author, 31 May 1995, Natal, transcript.
16. Informant 75, CAERN senior civil engineer and sewer construction coordinator, interview with author, 25 May 1995, Natal, transcript.
17. Informant 121, CAERN sewer construction division manager and former CAERN directorate member, interview with author, 1 June 1995, Natal, transcript; and Informant 122, CAERN staff member, interview with author, 7 June 1995, Natal, transcript.
18. Informant 122, CAERN construction division chief, interview by author, June 7 1995, Natal, transcript.
19. Informant 88, CAERN condominial sewer technician, interview with author, 11 May 1995, Natal, transcript.
20. Informant 78, CAERN sewer design division chief, interview with author, 24 May 1995, Natal, transcript.

21. Informant 75, CAERN senior civil engineer and sewer construction coordinator, interview with author, 24 May 1995, Natal, transcript.

22. Informant 75, CAERN senior civil engineer and sewer construction coordinator, interview with author, 25 May 1995, Natal, transcript.

23. Informant 99, Natal elected official, interview with author, 27 June 1995, Natal, transcript.

24. Informant 121, CAERN sewer construction division manager and former CAERN directorate member, interview with author, 1 June 1995, Natal, transcript.

25. Informant 121, CAERN sewer construction division manager and former CAERN directorate member, interview with author, 1 June 1995, Natal, transcript.

26. URBANA had to return the funds it did not use on the project.

27. Refer to chapter 7, Table 7-3 for a list of quotes from practitioners.

28. Informant 16, agency president, interview with author, 16 March 1995, Recife, transcript.

29. This result is based on the average response of five employees of the water and sanitation organization (i.e., CAERN) to the question, "How would you evaluate the overall performance of condominial sewers in Natal?" Possible answers were based on the following 5-point scale: 1-Poor, 2-Fair, 3-Good, 4-Very Good, 5-Excellent. The interviews were conducted in Natal in 1995.

30. Watson, 1995.

Chapter 5
Alignment and Influence in the City of Recife

Unlike Natal, the city of Recife embraced decentralization and began implementing condominial sewerage at the municipal level in 1985 using an *ad hoc* approach to service delivery. The city government implemented condominial sewer projects within a fragmented political environment, driven by Workers' Party political candidates in solidarity with activist engineers who believed in the merits of condominial sewerage. The success of individual projects in Recife seemed to depend on a perfect storm of events.

Three key themes characterize Recife's 1980–1995 innovation period. First, there was discontinuity in political support for condominial sewer projects from one administration to the next. Who was governor and who was mayor and whether or not they supported specific projects had an impact on the existence and performance of condominial sewer projects because mayors and governors set the development priorities and filled the implementing organizations with their employees. Second, there was not a single or universally agreed upon approach to the implementation of condominial sewers in Recife; rather, several different approaches were applied simultaneously by different organizations during the innovation period (i.e., an uncoordinated "ad hoc" approach). There were four implementing organizations in Recife, each using its own method that depended on the degree to which its engineering staff accepted condominial sewer technology and who had been elected to office. Political discontinuity and ad hoc implementation were signs of shifting alignment of interests among elected officials and implementing organizations. Third, residents mobilized their neighborhoods to make demands and exert influence on elected officials and implementing organizations, and to mobilize support for or against specific projects. Unlike Natal, community influence was a prominent feature of Recife's innovation period. Like the concept "alignment of interests," the concept "community influence" is introduced as convenient shorthand for a particular set of actions taken by residents on behalf of their condominial sewer projects.

Community Influence: Another Critical Concept

Influence is the persuasiveness that one entity is able to exert on another. In the case of Recife, individuals from a particular neighborhood exerted influence on behalf of their condominial sewer project, hence the term "community influence." Influence most often took the form of developing relationships with officials who had access to resources for condominial sewer projects. Individuals with personal, business, political, or familial relationships with public officials, sanitation staff, or politicians often have greater access to power holders and decision-makers and thus more potential influence. As explained by Mainwaring (1999), in Brazil "getting a job as a janitor in a public building, as a garbage collector, a teacher . . . frequently depends on political contacts."[1] The potential benefits of influence created by relationships and social ties can spread to the whole community when the ties are used in association with a neighborhood sanitation project.

Three state conditions contributed to a community's potential influence: the community's socio-economic status, the community's population size; and the extent that the community was organized. Condominial sewer practitioners in Recife and Natal reported that the socio-economic level of residents in the project area seemed to be associated with the performance of condominial sewer systems, and that project success was more difficult to achieve in poorer areas.[2] These statements match the tendencies described in the international development literature; that is, that there exist many challenges and biases against providing basic water and sanitation services to poor residents and that these challenges contribute to low coverage rates and poor performance.[3] One specific reason for worse performance was associated with the distribution of maintenance resources. Because the maintenance departments were routinely under-resourced, practitioners in Recife reported difficulties in meeting maintenance requirements across the city. Both routine maintenance and rehabilitation were subject to negotiation and influence, and because wealthier neighborhoods had more potential influence than poor neighborhoods, they tended to receive more frequent maintenance and rehabilitation, which contributed to their better performance.

Highly-populated communities tended to have more leverage than small communities because the larger population size represented the potential to deliver larger numbers of votes, a larger potential threat of mobilizing to make demands or to expose problems, and a relatively larger project impact. Collectively, these factors gave larger communities more potential influence on sanitation officials and politicians.

Communities that were effectively mobilized and organized also had more potential influence. Effective neighborhood organizations and grassroots popular movements became important during and following the democratic transition in Brazil, where neighborhoods first mobilized against the authoritarian military regime and then mobilized for "citizenship," which included the right to receive basic urban services.[4] Communities used the influence created by organizing and mobilizing to bring sanitation and other urban services into their neighborhood, and to improve the quality of service provided by public agencies.

The following sections describe the key events of Recife's condominial sewer innovation period. The period is discussed in four parts on the basis of the three conditions of potential community influence previously described. I divide Recife's experience from 1980 to 1995 into four periods, which are summarized in Table 5-1.

Pre-Implementation (1980–1984)

The early 1980s marked a turning point in Recife's water and sanitation sector, when the inability of the State Water and Sanitation Agency of Pernambuco (*Companhia Pernambucana de Saneamento*, or COMPESA) to implement its sewer plan or to expand sewer services to poor areas was broadly realized. In 1980, COMPESA issued the Recife Metropolitan Sewer Plan (Plan), which called for the expansion of conventional sewers in the three cities making up the Recife Metropolitan Region (RMR). COMPESA also proposed to use the *elo* (or water supply districts) as the standard service area for both water supply and sewage collection. According to COMPESA staff, the 1980 plan was never enacted because of the lack of staff, money, and equipment to maintain the public sewer, and because of internal resistance to the plan by senior staff. The municipal government had little confidence in COMPESA's ability to carry out the Plan because it considered conventional sewers to be infeasible; moreover, the City of Recife was interested in developing its own sanitation capability. The very next year, the municipal Urban Planning Agency (*Empresa de Planejamento Urbano do Recife*, or URB) revised the Recife portion of the Plan, replacing conventional sewers with condominial sewers.

This turning point was also marked by experimentation at many levels. While Recife's innovation period was still in the planning stages, condominial sewer research programs and pilot studies were already being conducted in Natal (Recife's regional neighbor) in the early 1980s. Full-scale condominial sewer projects were being implemented in other Northeast cities as well, and Brazil's professional engineering societies were beginning to disseminate information about condominial sewer technology. After this early period of research, pilot projects, and successful implementation outside of Recife, Recife started its own period of vigorous implementation of condominial sewers from 1985 to 1995.

Table 5-1. Timeline of events related to the implementation of condominial sewers in Recife from 1980 to 1995.

Year	Events
	Pre-Implementation
1980	COMPESA produces the Recife Metropolitan Sewer Plan covering three cities, four wastewater treatment plants, all with conventional sewers.
1981	URB revises the Recife portion of the Recife Metropolitan Sewer Plan, replacing conventional sewers with condominial sewers.
	Initiating Condominial Sewerage
1985	City agencies begin to install some of the first condominial sewers in Recife under the Condominial Program, the Condominial SOS Program, and the Recife Program.
1987	COHAB implements the Urbanization Program and the Habitation Program.
1988	Several completed condominial sewer systems are transferred from City agencies to COMPESA for ongoing maintenance.
	Revisiting Conventional Sewerage
1989	The Condominial Program is stopped by the newly-elected mayor. COMPESA constructs five condominial sewer projects during this phase, but does not perform regular maintenance on the City's condominial sewer projects.
1991	The Urbanization Program and the Habitation Program are stopped by the newly elected governor. Recife makes condominial sewers mandatory by adding them to municipal law under Lei No. 15.547/91.
1992	URB constructs four condominial projects in this period. COMPESA stops performing maintenance on some condominial sewer systems, but continues to collect the monthly fees.
	Consolidating Condominial Sewerage
1993	The newly elected mayor begins negotiations with COMPESA about their acceptance and maintenance of projects constructed by the City and issues the Director's Development Plan for the City of Recife, which establishes condominial sewers as the City's technical norm. City agencies are consolidated into a single condominial sewer implementing agency. URB implements three condominial sewer projects in this period.
1994	A new sewer plan (*Plano Estruturador de Esgotamento Sanitário do Recife*) calls for all planned increases in sewer coverage to use condominial technology. The Mayor proposes a new law (*Leis Complementares*) to resolve the political discontinuity problem in project implementation and to establish the roles and responsibilities of each implementing agency.

Sources: COMPESA, COHAB, EMLURB, and URB staff, interviews by author; 1994-1995, Recife, transcripts; http://www.recife.pe.gov.br/pr/galeria/index.php4; http://www.fundaj.gov.br/docs/pe/pe0036.html; and http://www.pernambuco.gov.br/governo_galeriadosgoves.htm.

Initiating Condominial Sewerage (1985–1988)

In 1985, Jarbas Vasconcelos of the centrist Party of the Brazilian Democratic Movement (PMDB) was elected Mayor of Recife. José Carlos Melo, the leading voice for condominial sewers in Brazil, was appointed Vice Mayor. This election marked the beginning of a surge of condominial sewer implementation in Recife. Prior to Mayor Jarbas (popular Brazilian politicians are commonly referred to by their first names), most of the condominial sewers in Pernambuco State were located outside of the capital city in small and medium-sized interior towns. In 1986, the City of Recife began to construct some of its first condominial sewers (in small-scale projects measured in the hundreds of connections per project) under the Condominial Program (*Projeto Condomínio*). From 1986 to 1989, the City Public Works Agency (*Empresa de Obras Públicas*, or OBRAS), located in the Secretary for Transportation and Public Works, served as the main implementing agency for condominial sewer projects supported by Mayor Jarbas and Vice Mayor Melo.

Vice Mayor Melo, also president of the AcquaPlan and Condominium Engineering Companies, was perhaps the most influential promoter of condominial sewer technology in Brazil. He brought to his hometown of Recife a wealth of condominial sewer experience, including experience installing condominial sewers in Natal with their State Water and Sanitation Agency (*Companhia de Águas e Esgotos do Rio Grande do Norte,* or CAERN), experience executing condominial sewers for state housing projects in interior towns with the Pernambuco State Housing Agency (*Companhia da Habitação,* or COHAB), and experience implanting condominial sewers throughout the Northeast region with the San Francisco River Hydroelectric Development Agency (*Companhia Hidro Eléctrica do São Francisco*, or CHESF). In addition to introducing Recife officials to the benefits of condominial sewers, Melo and his colleagues from CAERN taught many of Recife's city, state, and private engineers how to implement the new technology. Melo brought Edrise Aires, a former COMPESA employee and a defender of his ideas, into the City administration as President of OBRAS. President Edrise (also known by his first name) brought with him his loyal COMPESA staff.

Melo envisioned condominial sewers as an affordable alternative to conventional sewers.[5] He wanted to take advantage of the reduced overall costs associated with constructing sewers before installing pavement. He also wanted to eliminate the *dreno* system (described previously in chapter 3) and the general use of storm drains for sewage collection because of the resulting pollution problems and high volume of wastewater produced. Previously, conventional sewers had been sited based on the availability of an existing trunk sewer as a discharge point. Very few households were adjacent to an existing trunk sewer, and because COMPESA did not have the resources to extend the trunk sewer and treatment plant system the conventional sewer philosophy severely restricted any progress in sanitation.

The lack of sanitary sewerage was compounded by serious drainage problems in many areas of Recife. Ideally, drainage should be in place prior to the installation of sewers; otherwise residents would use their sewers for drainage, thereby exceeding the capacity of the system and creating performance problems.[6] On the other hand, installation of a drainage system prior to the sewer could potentially reduce demand for the sewer because residents would improperly use the drainage system as a sewer.[7]

During the mid-1980s in Recife, middle-income residents with well-functioning septic tanks were most interested in resolving pavement and drainage problems, not in resolving the sanitation problem.[8] Because of a general lack of demand for sewers among middle-income residents, Melo decided to attach condominial sewers to an existing City pavement program already being implemented by OBRAS. The existing pavement program from the previous mayoral administration was known by several names, including the Pavement Program (*Projeto para Pavimento*), the Program for Everyone (*Projeto para Todos*), and the One for All Program (*Projeto Um por Todos*).[9] Under this program, the City paved residential streets in partnership with residents. Neighborhoods had to show interest in the program by filling out a formal application. The City selected the most organized and most interested neighborhoods for pavement projects. Cobblestone pavement was the norm for most residential streets in Recife. Melo decided to focus on these interested neighborhoods because their streets were still unpaved (which facilitated sewer construction), and because they had already organized themselves to apply for a pavement project (which Melo considered advantageous). Under this new program, known as the Condominial Program, Melo proposed adding sewers as a condition of receiving pavement, and used community mobilization as a condition of program eligibility.

The Condominial Program included pavement and sewer services partly financed by the City and partly financed by residents. House connections and condominial sewers were installed under the Condominial Program; no public trunk sewers were installed because that was still COMPESA's role. Only those residents who agreed to pay for their house connection received a project. This led to some areas ending up with only a single street receiving sewer service. To be eligible to receive a project, residents had to mobilize, elect a representative, and express interest by completing a formal application for a project. These residents were added to the City's list of interested communities, and selected neighborhoods were offered a proposal for a sewer and pavement project. Unpaved streets that were already sewered by COMPESA were automatically included in the City's list because it was simple to install a condominial sewer and connect its discharge to COMPESA's public sewer.[10] Residents paid for the labor, and the City provided the construction materials. The criteria for deciding which middle-income areas would receive a project were as follows:[11]

- Areas with the most critical need for a sewer system;
- Areas with high interest and demand from residents;

- Residents willing to pay for the collective condominial sewer and individual house connections.

Under the Condominial Program, OBRAS installed about sixteen condominial sewer projects in middle-income neighborhoods. Eligibility requirements included consideration of need and consideration of resident demand for a project, and the OBRAS implementation approach included community participation. Working in collaboration with OBRAS, the City's Secretary for Social Action (*Secretaria Ação Social de Prefeitura*, or SAS) carried out the participation activities for OBRAS so that OBRAS could focus on the planning, design, construction, and maintenance activities. Backyard and front yard layouts were used in the majority of projects—use of the sidewalk layout was rare.

OBRAS administered a second condominial sewer program for poor residents at the same time it was administering the Condominial Program for middle-income residents. The Condomínio SOS Program (*SOS Condomínio*) was a City program funded through the Federal Secretary for Community Action (*Secretaria Especial de Ações Communitárias*) and implemented by OBRAS The program was created to provide total urbanization of favelas using participation during project implementation—the urbanization program included condominial sewer systems. In 1986, the municipal government had requested funds for this program from the Federal Bank of Brazil (*Caixa Econômica Federal*, or CEF) and in 1988 the funding arrived. OBRAS's criteria for deciding which poor areas of the city would receive an urbanization project were as follows:

- Areas with the most critical need for a sewer system;
- Areas in which more people could be served with the same amount of money;
- Areas without major technical problems (bad topography, no final destination, etc.);
- Areas where the residents were most interested in sewers.

Condomínio SOS staff visited all neighborhoods that requested a sewer system. They observed local conditions and the level of need for sewerage, and they held meetings with residents to determine what their priorities were in terms of infrastructure. There was a general lack of demand for sewers at that time because most residents wanted drainage under the widespread assumption that drainage would also resolve their sewage problem.[12] Condomínio SOS provided poor residents with an alternative to the traditional process of acquiring public assistance. The traditional process involved patron/client transactions in which politicians sought votes from poor residents in exchange for benefits that ranged from soccer team uniforms to small urban projects. One Condomínio SOS program official remarked that "all the poor areas with projects used this process, and poor areas without a link to politicians had no chance of getting a project."[13]

Electoral rules and term limits also had a direct impact on Condomínio SOS. Consecutive terms were not allowed, and the Jarbas administration would come to an end in 1989. However, because funds from CEF did not arrive until 1988, Condomínio SOS staff had less than one year to plan and implement its projects. As a result, many of its projects were not completed, and by the end of the Condomínio SOS Program only three neighborhoods were served with condominial sewers.

Another City agency, the Urban Planning Agency (*Empresa de Planejamento Urbano do Recife*, or URB), was simultaneously involved in implementing condominial sewers under a program called the Recife Program (*Projeto Recife*). The Recife Program was an infrastructure program financed by the National Housing Bank (*Banco Nacional da Habitação*, or BNH) with funds from the World Bank. The URB organization was parallel to OBRAS within the City hierarchy but was located in a different secretariat, the Secretary of Planning (*Secretaria de Planejamento*). URB was created to design, construct, and maintain infrastructure projects in poor areas known as special economic zones (*zeis*), whereas OBRAS at that time designed, constructed, and maintained infrastructure projects for the rest of the city.

The 1985–1988 period was marked by significant interagency struggle and role confusion between URB and OBRAS. Jaime Guzman was president of URB, and Teógenes Leitão served as URB's director of public works. President Guzman and many of the managers and engineers within URB did not completely agree with Melo's approach to condominial sewers. Unlike OBRAS, URB tended to implement condominial sewer projects without user participation. During this time, URB often competed for the same project areas as OBRAS using different sources of funding.

In 1987, Miguel Arraes was elected governor of the state of Pernambuco. Sharing the same centrist Party of the Brazilian Democratic Movement (PMDB) as Mayor Jarbas and running on a populist platform, Arraes's election initiated a peak period of political support for condominial sewer technology. Arraes's campaign was strongly supported at the grassroots level by poor and middle-income residents, who were now able to participate as citizens in Brazil's new democratic electoral process and political party system. The mobilization of votes was still often the only source of influence available to poor citizens, so many of these residents mobilized political support for Governor Arraes and ultimately received favela urbanization projects for their communities.

In one instance, poor residents started occupying (i.e., *invading*) a large vacant site in Recife for the purpose of establishing a community with urban services. The residents created an organization called the Occupation Commission (*Comissão de Ocupação*) to represent their interests, and hoped that newly elected Governor Arraes would provide them with urban services as he had done previously in other areas. The residents recalled that in the 1960s, during Arraes's first gubernatorial term, there had been a large invasion of poor citizens onto a vacant site and Arraes had legalized the land and provided infrastructure for the inhabitants. So when Arraes ran for office again in 1986, poor residents in Recife were betting on him giving them a project, and community leaders mobilized the inhabitants to "fight," actually to negotiate, for complete urbanization of the invaded area. Their mobilization tactics included assembling the votes of the community, developing a patron-client relationship, and negotiating with Arraes for the project. When Governor Arraes was elected, he included the invaded area in his favela urbanization program. Residents in this area also reported that politicians always visited their neighborhood just before election time.[14]

Arraes's new programs attempted to integrate favelas into cities by providing legal land tenure, by regularizing the layout of homes and streets, and by providing urban services (e.g., water, condominial sewerage, etc). Arraes started both the Habitation Program (*Projeto de Habitação),* a housing program implemented primarily outside of Recife, and the Urbanization Program (*Projeto de Urbanização*), a favela urbanization program (which included condominial sewers) that was implemented throughout the state and in Recife. Under these two state programs, large-scale projects (measured in thousands of connections per project) were implemented. Both of the Governor's programs were financed principally by CEF and were implemented through the Pernambuco State Housing Agency (*Companhia de Habitação*, or COHAB). Heavily subsidized favela urbanization projects were targeted to the very poor and included lots, water, sewerage, drainage, electricity, street lights, regrading, and pavement as necessary. The entire set of services was provided free to poor residents—only the monthly utility fees were charged. COHAB's implementation approach did not generally involve a formal participation program, although beneficiaries were usually expected to build their own homes after the urbanized lots were completed. Residents purchased their own building materials and either performed their own labor or hired contractors with their own funds. COHAB also installed condominial sewers in the interior of the state—also without formal participation—through its "*conjunto*" housing programs, and many poor residents who moved into COHAB homes without participation programs were not familiar with sewers or how to use them.[15]

To summarize the events of this period, condominial sewer technology was introduced into the city of Recife through four major programs: the Condominial Program (implemented by OBRAS with assistance from the *Secretaria Ação Social*), the Recife Program (implemented by URB), the Condomínio SOS Program (implemented by OBRAS), and the Urbanization Program (implemented by COHAB). Large-scale and small-scale condominial sewer projects were provided to poor, low-income, middle-income, and to a few high-income residents. The City agencies (OBRAS and URB) tended to concentrate on installing systems that either discharged to a public sewer or (more often) to the nearest available location, including the storm drain system. It is ironic that some condominial sewers ended up discharging to the storm drain system even though Melo's initial motivation for condominial sewers was to end reliance on the storm drain system for sewage collection. OBRAS embraced Melo's vision of condominial sewer technology and typically included participation programs in their projects. URB was more critical of the condominial approach and generally did not embrace the participation component.

The main role of the State agencies (COMPESA and COHAB) was to install public trunk sewers, so that there would be something for the condominial sewers to connect to. In addition, COMPESA was responsible (theoretically) for maintaining all sewer systems and for administering water and sewer utility billing. Neither COMPESA nor COHAB embraced participation for the majority of their projects, and COMPESA was generally critical of condominial sewer design standards and construction quality. One practitioner estimated that up to 80 percent of the engineers in COMPESA were opposed to condominial sewer technology during this time period.[16] EMLURB staff estimated that COMPESA accepted maintenance responsibility for approximately 60 percent of the City's condominial sewer connections (not including projects that were not completed); the remaining 40 percent of the connections were left without a formal maintenance agency.[17]

Revisiting Conventional Sanitation (1989–1992)

Joaquim Francisco of the rightist Party of the Liberal Front (PFL) took office as Mayor of Recife in 1989. He appointed José de Anchieta dos Santos to replace Edrise Aires as the president of OBRAS. Edrise Aires moved to COMPESA with his entire OBRAS staff, including the coordinator of the Condominial Program. The coordinator of Condomínio SOS also left OBRAS after disagreeing with the Francisco administration's non-participation approach to her program. José Carlos Melo left his position as Vice Mayor of Recife to become the State Secretary of Sanitation for the Governor Arraes administration. In his new position, Melo was able to direct condominial sewer funding to the interior city of Petrolina under Brazil's Medium-Size Cities Program (*Cidades de Porte Médio*).

No unfinished condominial sewer projects from the previous administration were completed by the Mayor Francisco administration. The Condominial Program was paralyzed by the new mayor, who was not interested in promoting the programs of the previous administration. Such discontinuity and political individualism were common practice throughout Brazil (as previously discussed), and could be considered a manifestation of Brazil's history of political patronage, clientelism, and executive privilege. Because projects and programs were often designed to serve a particular clientele (e.g., a particular neighborhood), newly elected officials had no sense of obligation for maintaining the previous official's projects and programs. On the contrary, the newly elected official had his or her own clientele to consider. The very logic of patronage and clientelism precluded continuity from one regime to the next. Francisco continued to spend the funds remaining from the previous administration to build projects, but he eliminated the participation component and focused only on the public parts of the system (not condominial sewers and house connections). In the case of one condominial sewer project, Francisco completed the public trunk sewer but did not complete the condominial sewer or house connections. The result was a functioning public trunk sewer system with few or no homes connected to it.

By 1989, OBRAS had completed several condominial sewer projects and had transferred the maintenance responsibility over to COMPESA. However, COMPESA did not perform regular maintenance duties on all of these projects even though users continued to pay sewer fees to COMPESA. Ostensibly, COMPESA used a two-step process for deciding whether or not to accept responsibility for maintenance on condominial sewers implemented by the City agencies. Prior to construction, COMPESA would form a three-member committee—made up of one representative each from COMPESA's Engineering, Construction, and Maintenance Departments—to review the implementing agency's design and write a report that included design recommendations. After the implementing agency constructed the project, COMPESA would form another committee to review the as-built drawings and to determine whether or not COMPESA should accept maintenance responsibility for the project. Reasons for not accepting maintenance responsibility included a lack of as-built drawings, lack of an appropriate sewage destination, or a design that did not meet COMPESA guidelines. Some projects were initially accepted and then subsequently abandoned by COMPESA. Reasons given by COMPESA staff for system abandonment included poor project performance, excessive maintenance costs, or substandard design. Although the results of these design and acceptance reviews were documented in agency memoranda and letters, there were no formal written rules, criteria, or norms for acceptance or abandonment.[18] In deciding whether to accept maintenance responsibilities on a project, COMPESA staff used so-called "practical rules." For example, condominial sewer projects would not be accepted by COMPESA unless the following technical criteria were satisfied:

- Mandatory use of iron-trimmed manhole covers;
- Maximum distances between manholes ≤ 80 meters;
- Standard dimensions for manholes;
- Minimum diameters for pump suction piping;
- Minimum distances between pumps and overhead structures.

It should be mentioned that some of these practical rules were often violated by definition, because condominial technology required relaxed design standards in order to make sewerage more affordable to people who were left unserved by conventional design standards. Over and above these so-called practical rules, COMPESA staff acknowledged that the decision to accept maintenance responsibility for a project was also a political decision, because the neighborhoods that received projects had already been chosen on political grounds by higher officials.[19] It was, therefore, probably no coincidence that COMPESA, under Governor Arraes, did not agree to maintain Mayor Francisco's condominial sewer projects. During this time, the mayor and the governor were politically opposed, so their implementing agencies had little incentive to cooperate.

State sewer projects continued to be implemented with state money and with funds from the World Bank via the Grand Recife Program (*Projeto Grande Recife*), which was a continuance of the previous Recife Program. These funds were channeled from the World Bank to CEF, through the Municipal Development Foundation (*Fundação de Desenvolvimento Municipal*, or FIDEM), and down to the Pernambuco state government. The earlier Recife Program, which had a stronger focus on condominial sewers, was also funded by the World Bank during the 1980s, but its funds had been channeled directly to the City government in an attempt to reduce the impact of corruption.[20]

Governor Arraes's Urbanization and Habitation Programs continued to be implemented by COHAB until 1991, when Joaquim Francisco left his position as Mayor of Recife to take office as Governor of the state. As expected, Francisco eliminated the Urbanization and Habitation Programs and fired about one hundred COHAB employees who had been associated with these programs and who were aligned with former Governor Arraes. The fired employees went back to work for their "home" government agencies in the Recife municipal government (such as URB) and in other counties and cities. Francisco's Vice Mayor, Gilberto Marques Paulo (also of the rightist PFL party), took over as Mayor of Recife from 1990 to 1992. He appointed Roberto Andrade as president of OBRAS in 1990. After 1990, with Francisco as Governor and his ally as Mayor of Recife, COMPESA showed little interest in Recife's condominial sewers. COMPESA did not even allow condominial sewer-related documents into its archives, and much of COMPESA's pre-1991 condominial sewer data were destroyed.[21]

Consolidating Condominial Sewerage (1993–1995)

In 1993, Jarbas was re-elected to his second mayoral term, this time without a party affiliation but continuing with his populist platform. The Pernambuco Daily Newspaper announced that, for the second time, Jarbas had been voted best mayor in all of Brazil in a public survey.[22] His approval rating was over 70 percent, the highest in the country at that time.

Jarbas continued working on the unfinished condominial sewer projects that had been started during his first term. City condominial sewer staff continued to criticize COMPESA for not performing maintenance on many condominial sewer systems while continuing to collect tariffs on the systems. Jarbas initiated the Plan of Order (*Plano de Ordenamento de 1994*) to formalize his negotiations with COMPESA about their acceptance and maintenance of projects constructed by the City. Jarbas wanted to transform informal maintenance agreements into law so that COMPESA could be relied upon to maintain City projects. In the case of failed negotiations with COMPESA, Jarbas planned to develop a permanent maintenance group within the City that would last beyond his political tenure. This option would be less desirable, however, because the City would have to acquire the resources, equipment, and staff to perform the maintenance.

Jarbas also reinforced his decentralized, micro-regional approach to sewer collection and treatment by issuing the Director's Plan for the Development of Recife (*Plano Diretor de Desenvolvimento da Cidade do Recife*) and by including the text of a little known condominial sewer law (Lei 15.547/91) into Article 77 of the Plan. This Plan represented a direct challenge to COMPESA's regional sewage collection and centralized treatment approach because the Plan attempted to institutionalize condominial sewer technology by a) mandating condominial sewers (not conventional sewers) as the technical norm for the City, and b) stating that residents were responsible for the maintenance of their sewer connection. Jarbas's persistence in pushing for an innovative approach to sewerage in Recife contributed to a sense of hope and possibility among many sewer practitioners. In his first term, Jarbas had proved he could expand sewer service in Recife using condominial sewer technology implemented by municipal agencies. At the same time, COMPESA had shown an inability to expand conventional sewer service in Recife for the previous fifteen years. The following statement by a condominial sewer practitioner exemplifies the promise attributed to Jarbas's condominial approach:

> "The sewer law (Lei 15.547/91) and the *Ordenamento* mean that everyone in Recife will eventually be served by condominial sewers." (Informant 1, engineering consultant, interview by author, 2 March 1995, Recife, transcript)

Mayor Jarbas made some key organizational improvements in his second term. He moved URB from the Secretary of Planning into the Secretary of Infrastructure (previously called the Secretary of Transportation and Public Works) with OBRAS. He also changed the name and responsibilities of OBRAS to eliminate the apparent overlap in duties between the two organizations. OBRAS's name was changed to the Urban Cleanup Agency (*Empresa Municipal de Limpeza Urbana*, or EMLURB), and its previous responsibilities for planning, design, and construction were moved to URB. The new EMLURB agency was temporarily tasked with administering maintenance for condominial sewer projects of all sizes (through contracts with private firms), performing small sewer system rehabilitation and reconstruction (less than three hundred connections), evaluating condominial sewer projects, and surveying and mapping existing condominial sewer projects so that reliable as-built information could be made available (which would improve the chances of COMPESA accepting City projects). EMLURB was also the agency that, if necessary, would become the City's official sewer maintenance agency if negotiations with COMPESA were not successful.

EMLURB no longer had responsibility for the design and construction of condominial sewer projects as it had when it was called OBRAS. URB now served as the single implementing agency for new condominial project construction and was the main agency involved in discussions with COMPESA about establishing clear maintenance roles and responsibilities. Under Jarbas's new organization scheme for City agencies, only the URB agency performed new project design, construction, and participation. URB was also responsible for large system rehabilitation and reconstruction (projects with more than three hundred connections).

URB's implementation approach for condominial sewers changed dramatically in this time period, as the agency took into account the lessons learned from the previous Jarbas term. The organization had now embraced the participatory approach. One practitioner remarked that "engineers now believe that the education, orientation, and mobilization of residents is needed and important. This is the biggest change."[23] Under its new approach, URB implemented condominial sewers in the following four general approaches, depending on the income of neighborhood served:

1. For middle-income and high-income neighborhoods, the residents who wanted a sewer connection decided on which layout they preferred (backyard, sidewalk, or front yard), they paid 100 percent of the capital costs (materials and labor), and they either contracted out the construction of their house connections or did it themselves. The City constructed the condominial sewer. For backyard and front yard systems, residents were responsible for maintaining private house connections and collective condominial sewers. For sidewalk systems, COMPESA or the City was responsible for maintaining the sidewalk sewer.

2. For low-income neighborhoods, the residents who wanted a sewer connection decided on which of the three layouts they preferred, and they paid for the capital cost of materials for their house connections. The City constructed the condominial sewer and house connections. For backyard and front yard systems, residents were responsible for maintaining private house connections and collective condominial sewers. For sidewalk systems, COMPESA or the City was responsible for maintaining the sidewalk sewer.

3. For poor and very poor neighborhoods, the residents who wanted a sewer connection received only backyard condominial systems (no layout choice was offered), and they paid 50 percent of the capital cost of materials for their house connections and bathroom. The City constructed the condominial sewer and house connections. Residents were responsible for maintaining private house connections and collective condominial sewers.

4. In favelas, the residents who wanted a sewer connection received only backyard condominial systems (no layout choice was offered), and they constructed their own bathrooms using materials provided by the City. The City constructed the condominial sewer and house connections, and provided bathroom materials. Residents were responsible for maintaining private house connections and collective condominial sewers.

By 1995, the City of Recife was planning larger-scale condominial sewer projects, such as one proposal to serve 500,000 residents in the flat center of the city, which was only 10 percent sewered. In cases where COMPESA did not accept maintenance responsibility for a project, the City was now tentatively accepting maintenance responsibility through its EMLURB agency.

Changes were also taking place at the state level. In November 1994, after winning the gubernatorial election under the leftist Brazilian Socialist Party (PSB), Arraes invited all of "his employees" back to their old jobs at COHAB through an ad in the Vida Urbana section of the Pernambuco Daily (*Diáro de Pernambuco*) newspaper. Since his previous 1987–1990 term as governor, Arraes had fallen out with Jarbas Vasconcelos, had left his old party (the centrist PMDB), and had gained the support of the leftist PSB political party. Arraes began his 1995–1998 term as governor at the first of the year in 1995, having won again on a populist platform.

During the 1980s, COMPESA had not been very interested or involved in the implementation of condominial sewers in the city of Recife. The agency was, by and large, resistant to using participation in the planning, design, and construction of condominial sewers, and had been generally opposed to accepting the maintenance responsibility for condominial sewers implanted by City agencies. At the same time that it had actively resisted condominial sewers in Recife, COMPESA had been more involved with implementing condominial sewers outside of the capital city, such as in the interior city of Petrolina. But by 1995, COMPESA's attitude toward condominial sewers in Recife changed dramatically, as expressed in the following statement by a COMPESA engineer:

> The attitude of COMPESA toward condominial sewers has improved greatly, with more knowledge, more acceptance of systems, and agreement now with the technology. If COMPESA had the money, we would probably prefer conventional sewers, but the reality is we do not have money and have therefore grown to accept condominial sewers. (Informant 12, COMPESA engineer, interview by author, 10 March 1995, Recife, transcript.)

I believe COMPESA's limited access to direct funding, combined with the *Plano Diretor* which institutionalized condominial sewer technology as the norm in the city of Recife had a lot to do with COMPESA's evolution. The organization faced the option of either evolving or remaining on the sidelines. COMPESA staff noted two problems with the *Plano Diretor*, however. First, the Plan only applied to the city of Recife while the City's sewer system extended beyond the city limits to surrounding cities that were also served by COMPESA. Second, compliance with the Plan was difficult when one neighbor cut off, cemented in, or otherwise sabotaged the collective condominial sewer system.[24] Nevertheless, the Plan was put into effect despite its imperfections. In 1995, COMPESA's Alternative Technology Program began to implement condominial sewers in Recife under the PROSANEAR Program (funded by the World Bank).[25] COMPESA was also initiating a participation and education component that would be implemented statewide through a permanent staff of social workers.[26] And COMPESA was doing maintenance on some condominial sewer systems, particularly those systems located in influential communities such as the favela that had been urbanized under the state's Urbanization Program. That community had remained well-organized after their project was completed; it had an active neighborhood association and a strong president. The president reported that he made monthly visits to COMPESA, in person, to voice complaints on behalf of his neighborhood and to reinforce the need for continued maintenance of their condominial sewer system and other infrastructure.

Alignment and Influence as Elements of Performance

This chapter has presented the specific conditions of condominial sewer emergence in the City of Recife from 1980 to 1995. Unlike Natal, there was no long period of coherent implementation during Recife's innovation period. Alignments were constantly shifting, communities had differing degrees of influence, and performance was highly mixed from the beginning to the end of the period. During the 1980–1995 period in Recife, alignments between elected officials and implementing organizations were generally unstable at both the municipal and state levels. Characteristics of Recife's implementing environment at that time included regime discontinuity, lack of inter-agency cooperation, lack of consistent support for condominial sewer technology and participation, and an inconsistent response to popular needs for basic sanitation.[27] As a result, successful performance was uncommon and tended to depend on both the alignment of interests among officials and the influence of communities on officials (elected and appointed). A key point expressed by many of Recife's condominial sewer practitioners was that participation in all aspects of project implementation mattered greatly.[28] Nevertheless, participation was not consistently applied, and even when it was, unpredictable changes in the alignments of politicians and organizations appeared to have an overwhelming impact on condominial sewer project performance. In addition, the fact that neighborhoods received service according to their level of influence was a second overwhelming factor in project performance.

One indication of performance is the number of sewer connections; however, it is difficult to state with accuracy the number of conventional and condominial sewer connections in Recife during the period of innovation. Total sewer connections can be roughly estimated by the number of dwelling units billed (known as *economías* in COMPESA's R12 computerized billing records). In 1994, COMPESA billing records showed 40,427 conventional sewer units billed and 10,272 condominial sewer units billed. However, the actual number of connections was greater than the number of dwelling units billed, so an accurate estimate of the total number of household sewer connections is difficult to obtain. For example, single-family households with condominial sewers were typically billed as individual dwelling units even when the homes shared a collective block sewer. Apartment complex owners were typically billed for one dwelling unit and an entire building was counted as one sewer connection, even though multiple dwelling units (or households) were served. A high-level

COMPESA official estimated that in 1995 there were on the order of 20,000 condominial connections in Recife.[29] It is possible to obtain a more accurate estimate of the total number of water connections for residential, commercial, industrial, and public customers because all dwelling units are billed individually for water service. In 1994, the number of water units billed in Recife was 227,370. Census data indicate that by 1994 only 24 percent of the 1.3 million people in Recife had access to sewers (not including septic tanks).

As of 1995, Recife had a sketchy overall record of condominial sewer project performance. Fully half of the forty-three condominial sewer projects implemented in Recife from 1980 to 1995 had less than fifty connections each. Many condominial sewer projects were never concluded, a large percentage of projects barely functioned, and most projects were not designed with a suitable destination for the collected sewage.[30] There were some successful projects; however, agency staff I interviewed unanimously characterized Recife's overall performance as "fair" when choosing among the categories "bad," "fair," "good," "very good," and "excellent."[31] The following quotes from practitioners in Recife provide additional characterizations of condominial sewer performance in Recife as of 1995:[32]

> The number of functioning projects is very small.
>
> Some [projects] are very bad, some are good.
>
> Sanitation is bad here in Recife.

These characterizations are supported by the findings of a separate survey of condominial sewer experience commissioned by the World Bank in 1993.[33] The study investigated and compared the condominial sewer experiences of seven Brazilian cities: Brasília, Recife, Natal, Cuiabá, Joinville, Petrolina, and Itapissuma. The sample of cities chosen for the investigation consisted of two-thirds of all known condominial sewer connections at that time: 52,550 out of 75,000 total connections. In the study, the overall record of condominial sewer performance in Recife was characterized as "bad," based on a three-category scale of excellent/good/bad.[34] The study found that some projects were operating well even in the badly performing cities of Recife and Cuiabá, and that all cities had some problems.[35]

Recife's innovation period represented a wide range of approaches implemented at full-scale (with a few pilot-scale projects within them), but this was not the result of a planned demonstration of these approaches. Rather, the wide range of approaches was symptomatic of a context characterized by intense multiplicity, including: 1) various simultaneous approaches to sanitation development; 2) lack of collaboration and even conflicts among multiple sanitation organizations; 3) implementation of projects in neighborhoods with multiple socio-economic levels, population sizes, and potential influence; and 4) unpredictable alignment of interests among elected officials and implementing organizations.

Closing Remarks for Chapter 5

Chapter 5 has described how condominial sewerage became established in Recife, the second Northeast capital city to adopt the innovation. Although located in the same region as Natal, Recife offered a very different urban setting. The degree of decentralized governance in the sanitation sector and the influence of organized communities in Recife led to very different outcomes compared to Natal's innovation period. Recife is a story of battles between competing regimes over how sanitation services should be delivered, what role communities should have in that delivery, and whether or how poor communities could be included in the service. The chapter explored the complicated relations between politicians, engineers, and citizens involved in sanitation development, and explained how isolated successes emerged from (or in spite of) these relations. Urban development in Recife was much more complicated and success much more difficult to attain because of the difficulty in forming and maintaining stable project support coalitions.

Thus far the analysis of condominial sewerage in Natal and Recife has traced the movements of three actors: elected officials, implementing organizations, and (to a lesser degree) communities. Recife's experience raises questions about the relationship between the alignment of interests, the influence of communities, and project performance; questions such as the direction or form of causality and whether the intense multiplicity of actors was the result of healthy experimentation, complete dysfunction, or something in between. In an attempt to answer the questions raised thus far, the next chapter introduces a new actor—the projects—and traces the making of project performance in greater detail.

Notes

1. Mainwaring, 1999, 182.
2. For example, Informant 1, engineering consultant, former Recife official, and former state official, Interview by author, 1 December 1994, Recife, transcript; and Informant 76, CAERN social worker, Interview by author, May 5, 1995, Natal, transcript.
3. Menendez, 1991; and Solo et al., 1993.
4. Hochstetler, 2000; and Mainwaring, 1989.
5. Jose Carlos Melo, personal communication with author, March 1995, Recife.
6. Jose Carlos Melo, personal communication with author, March 1995, Recife.
7. Jose Carlos Melo, personal communication with author, March 1995, Recife.
8. Informant 1, engineering consultant and former official, interview by author, 2 March 1995, Recife, transcript.
9. Informant 3, EMLURB official, interview by author, March 13, 1995, Recife, transcript; and Informant 16, president of a Recife sewer agency, interview by author, March 16, 1995, Recife, transcript.
10. Informant 16, president of a Recife sewer agency, interview by author, March 16, 1995, Recife, transcript.

11. Informant 4, URB social scientist and former project director in the Secretary for Social Action, interview by author, March 14, 1995, Recife, transcript.

12. Informant 3, EMLURB official, interview by author, March 13, 1995, Recife, transcript.

13. Informant 3, EMLURB official, interview by author, March 13, 1995, Recife, transcript.

14. Nance, 2004, 515–16.

15. Informant 16, president of a Recife sewer agency, interview by author, March 16, 1995, Recife, transcript.

16. Informant 31, consulting engineer and former director of a state agency, interview by author, 3 March 1995, Recife, transcript.

17. Informant 9, EMLURB engineer, interview by author, March 8, 1995, Recife, transcript.

18. Informant 12, COMPESA engineer, interview by author, March 10, 1995, Recife, transcript.

19. Informant 29, COMPESA technical manager, interview by author, March 16, 1995, Recife, transcript.

20. Corruption had (and still has) a tremendous impact on Brazil's ability to make effective use of public monies, and it was widely perceived to exist on every level of the Brazilian government. The World Bank attempted to reduce the impact of corruption by reducing the number of institutions through which Recife Program money had to flow. In this case, funds went as directly as possible to municipal governments.

21. Informant 3, EMLURB official, interview by author, March 13, 1995, Recife, transcript.

22. *Diario de Pernambuco*, January 8, 1995.

23. Informant 9, EMLURB engineer, interview by author, March 8, 1995, Recife, transcript.

24. Informant 12, COMPESA engineer, interview by author, March 10, 1995, Recife, transcript.

25. Informant 12, COMPESA engineer, interview by author, March 10, 1995, Recife, transcript; and direct knowledge of the PROSANEAR program obtained while working as a summer intern at the World Bank Water and Sanitation Division, Washington, DC, 1993 and 1994.

26. Informant 12, COMPESA engineer, interview by author, March 10, 1995, Recife, transcript.

27. Refer to chapter 5 for evidence supporting this statement.

28. Refer to chapter 7 for quotes from practitioners.

29. Informant 37, COMPESA technical director, interview by author, November 23, 1994, Recife, transcript.

30. Informant 16, president of a Recife sewer agency, interview by author, March 16, 1995, Recife, transcript.

31. This result is based on the average response of eight agency employees to the question, "How would you evaluate the overall performance of condominial sewers in Recife?" Possible answers were based on the following 5-point scale: 1-Poor, 2-Fair, 3-Good, 4-Very Good, 5-Excellent. The interviews were conducted in Recife in the month of March, 1995.

32. Informant 16, president of a Recife sewer agency, interview by author, March 16, 1995, Recife, transcript; Informant 59, COMPESA division chief, interview by au-

thor, March 20, 1995, Recife, transcript; and Informant 100, president of an engineering company, interview by author, 19 March 1995, Recife, transcript.

33. Watson, 1993.

34. The seven cities represented sixty neighborhoods; however, cities were the unit of analysis, so there was no evaluation of individual projects. Also, there was no description of how the excellent/good/bad performance measures were derived.

35. Watson, 1993, 21.

Chapter 6
An Actor-Oriented Account of Condominial Sewerage

Thus far I have mentioned how people in Brazil used collective action to organize their neighborhoods and exert community influence for the purpose of obtaining basic urban services, including condominial sewers. People negotiated with elected officials for inclusion of their neighborhoods in the distribution of basic urban services, and they made collective demands on implementing organizations for maintenance and rehabilitation of their neighborhood infrastructure. I have also introduced some of the ways people participated in condominial sewer programs under the direction of an implementing organization. In this chapter I will illustrate in detail how coalitions of different actors emerged in specific projects, and I will use these results as the basis for a situated understanding of why some projects performed better than others. To protect the privacy of individual residents who lived in the study areas, projects in Natal will be identified as N1, N2, etc., and projects in Recife will be identified as R1, R2, etc.

Identifying the Actors

This chapter will focus on the actions and associations of four categories of actors directly involved in condominial sewer projects in Natal and Recife during the innovation period (1980–1995): projects, residents, agencies, and officials. Residents in the project area who participated in mobilizing and decision-making activities interacted primarily with each other, with the employees of implementing agencies, and in some cases with elected and appointed officials. Residents who participated in construction and maintenance activities interacted directly with each other and with the physical components of the project. Implementing agencies (i.e., the employees and their agents or contractors) had direct interactions with all projects through planning and design decisions and construction and maintenance work (with or without participation from residents in these activities). Appointed and elected officials interacted with each other, with the employees of implementing agencies, and with the communities they served (especially with community leaders). Each actor is described in turn below.

Projects

Projects that are made to operate as planned and to produce desired benefits are generally judged in terms of their relative performance, while projects that fail to achieve these advantages are usually abandoned and forgotten as if they did not even exist. Failed and abandoned projects leave few traces of their presence, while successful projects leave a constant stream of evidence that indicates their degree of performance at any given time. If people connected to the project perceive that performance is declining, then the people who can ensure the project's survival will either restore the project or they will allow the project to die—to fall into disrepair, eventual abandonment, and non-existence. Thus, a project can be seen to hold a relative state of existence, measurable by the set of tracings left by its degree of presence in the world. To observe these tracings for condominial sewer projects, I made field observations of as many aspects of the physical system as possible. These included transect walks of the area served by the system and inspections of the condition of pipes, cleanout boxes, tanks, layouts, and environmental conditions. I also conducted in-depth interviews with as many of the people connected to the project as possible. These included people who lived in the project area; practitioners involved in project planning, design, construction, and maintenance; employees of the water and sanitation organizations who oversaw the project delivery process; and officials who helped bring the project to fruition. This wide range of information about a project's state of existence will be consolidated into the concept "performance," measured as an index on an ordinal scale from 0 (representing complete failure) to 100 (the highest possible achievement on all measures).[1]

Residents

The residents connected to the project include people who lived in the project area; people who served as representatives of the project area; people who participated in the project; people whose homes were physically linked to the project by way of fixtures, pipes, and fittings; and people who used the project to meet their sanitation needs whether or not they were physically connected. I conducted in-depth interviews (lasting up to sixty minutes each) with random samples of residents for each individual project, and in some neighborhoods I also conducted group interviews (i.e., focus groups).

Agencies

A range of organizations was engaged in the implementation of condominial sewer projects in Natal and Recife. Most common were state-owned water and sanitation companies, municipal urban planning and public works departments, state housing agencies, engineering firms, construction companies, and individual contractors. Within these organizations were key individuals—agency staff—who had played central roles on condominial sewer project teams or working groups and who knew individual projects more thoroughly than anyone else. These practitioners were most often engineers, social scientists, and maintenance operators and technicians, but they also included architects, planners, and other disciplines. I conducted numerous in-depth interviews with the key practitioners of each project studied; I spent months with them in their offices, read their files, gathered their documents, and compiled their data; I accompanied them on site visits; and I attended participation meetings they convened in the communities.

Officials

Government officials involved in condominial sewer projects may be elected or appointed. Elected officials included mayors, vice mayors, and governors; appointed officials included the directors and managers of city and state agencies (e.g., water and sanitation, planning, housing, public works, etc.), and the project directors of the various condominial sewers programs. I did not have direct access to governors, but I was able to hold one-on-one interviews with the mayor of Natal, the former vice mayor of Recife; the former secretary of sanitation of Pernambuco, and the directors of the engineering, planning, and maintenance departments at CAERN, COMPESA, URB, and EMLURB, and all of the program managers associated with the selected projects.[2]

Tracing the Network of Associations

Condominial sewer technology was created for the purpose of extending basic sanitation service into areas that were unserved by conventional sanitation. Most unserved areas were poor and low income, but in practice the technology was applied to neighborhoods at all income levels. The seven projects I selected for in-depth study covered five income categories: poor (R3), low income (R2, N2), lower middle income (N3), middle income (R1), and high income (N1, N4) (these categories were defined previously in Table 3-1). I will begin in poor and low-income neighborhoods to observe the emergence of the new technology in some of the most difficult settings, and will follow with a discussion of the remaining neighborhoods for comparative purposes. This set of selected projects is not representative. These projects were selected because local practitioners identified them as among the best or worst experiences of participation and performance in their respective cities, and I expected to learn the most from a set of polar projects.

Project R3

Project R3 was partially introduced in the previous chapter. Residents in the area developed a patron-client relationship with a newly elected governor and received an urbanization project. The project was installed in a favela in the hills of Recife between 1987 and 1990 as part of Pernambuco State's *Projeto Urbanizacao* program under Governor Miguel Arraes. The project included complete urbanization of the favela, including planned and regraded lots, pavement, drainage, water supply, electricity, street sewers, condominial sewers, community septic tanks, sewage pump stations, final discharge to a nearby river (*Rio Morno*), and new homes constructed by the residents. Residents subsequently turned some of the lots into stores and schools, which were not included in the project design. The project was planned and funded through COHAB and was accepted and successfully transferred to COMPESA after completion. COHAB hired a large engineering and construction contractor to design and construct the public services (water supply, street sewers and condominial sewers, drainage canals, pavement, electricity, etc.). Approximately 95 percent of the project was completed within one political term. At the time of the fieldwork (1995), 100 percent of the sampled residents were connected to the condominial sewer, and performance was among the best in Recife. COMPESA provided regular maintenance of the public street sewer, while residents were expected to perform maintenance within their lots. Photo 6-1 shows a street scene and the typical condition of the neighborhood in 1994–1995, five years after the project had been completed.

COHAB conducted a participation program with respect to the improvement of housing lots. Although COHAB's participation program primarily focused on the housing aspect of the project, the program also instructed residents on how to build house connections and how to use the sewer system. COHAB provided construction materials and money for residents to use to build their homes and house connections, and residents signed a contract to repay COHAB over a twenty-five-year period. During and after construction, as much as 30 percent of the construction materials were stolen by poor residents for resale. Turnover was high during implementation as many residents sold their lots or homes to new residents. Other implementation difficulties included an inconsistent

See photo 6-1 in photospread at the end of this chapter.

water supply (by January 1995, the area still only received six hours of water service every other day) and a lack of reliable project financing (however, practitioners reported that they experienced financing problems on every project). The project's pump station was only partially finished because of a change of governor at the end of the project construction period. COMPESA employees were present during construction, they evaluated the design of the project, and they eventually accepted the project as part of the city sewer system. As new residents moved into the area, they requested connection to the sewer system from COMPESA. This growth put higher demands on the sewage system, especially the pumps.

Residential lots were constructed by creating a series of long plateaus on steep hills and by developing regular blocks in the flatter areas and hilltops. A main sewer collection pipe was constructed on each plateau before homes were built. Because of the variety of topography in the area, some lots were interconnected with backyard condominial sewers, and others had sidewalk condominial or individual connections to the street sewer. In most cases, COHAB selected the layout of the condominial sewers and the location of the cleanout boxes on individual lots, and when residents arrived, these were already built. In cases where they were not already built, residents and COHAB field crews worked together to lay out and construct the onsite portion of the system, depending on the interest and skill level of the resident. COHAB held project meetings and showed educational videos to residents, but as the project was finished in one area after another the sewer system experienced numerous blockages. COHAB personnel believed some residents did not know how to use the system. Social workers from COHAB were then brought in to educate the residents on the use of the sewer system. This education was done through house-to-house visits and distribution of pamphlets.

Project R3 residents participated in four categories of project participation: mobilizing, decision-making, construction, and maintenance. Residents expressed great interest in the project by organizing and mobilizing autonomously prior to the project. There was little or no resident involvement in the water, sewer, and drainage parts of the urbanization project, since these services were being provided by COHAB while the residents were constructing their homes. The residents had little or no input in decisions regarding the layout and construction of the condominial sewer; this reduced level of participation may be attributed to the large-scale and multiple objectives of this project. However, many residents did make layout and construction decisions with regard to their house connections and onsite piping. Project R3 residents also exhibited a high level of participation in maintenance, with residents taking responsibility for onsite problems such as blockages. In addition, community leaders took the initiative to make demands on COMPESA staff with regard to ongoing maintenance of the public parts of the system. Consequently, when the sewer system became plugged or needed maintenance, COMPESA reliably resolved the problem and the system continued to function (as of 1995). The project achieved an extremely high connection rate, high perceived beneficial impacts, and relatively high levels of satisfaction, all contributing to a relatively high performance score of 71 (on an ordinal scale from 0 to 100). This project was considered among the best performing condominial sewer projects in Recife at the time of the field-work.

The main point to take away from Project R3 is that condominial sewer implementation was a function of the residents' ability to affect the course of events in their neighborhood. Residents were actively engaged in project activities, comprised of participation in project construction, project maintenance, project mobilizing, and project decision-making. Community participation in construction and maintenance (C&M) included contributions of residents' time, money, and labor for project construction and maintenance. Project R3 residents assisted in some aspects of sewer construction on their lots; however, their contributions toward maintenance of the private parts of the system was widespread. Community participation in mobilizing and decision-making (M&D) included residents mobilizing to learn about and foster support for the project and residents' involvement in project decisions. Project R3 residents mobilized quite well to participate in the project; however, their involvement in condominial sewer decisions was limited by the implementing organization.

Despite their poverty (i.e., Project R3 residents were classified as poor on the basis of average household income, as defined in Table 3-1), this community developed the ability to effectively communicate their interests and the influence to persuade politicians and implementing organizations to take their interests into account in ways that contributed to a successful condominial sewer project. The population size of the project area (approximately 6,340 people—very high compared to other condominial sewer projects in Recife at that time), the relatively high degree of organization actually achieved by the residents, and the demonstrated effectiveness of the community leaders' actions all likely contributed to the realization of community influence. Project R3 was also fortunate to have been implemented during a period in which the interests between elected officials and implementing organizations were aligned in support of the project. The project was implemented by a single state-level organization, COHAB, that supported condominial sewer technology in general (although it was less supportive of participation, per se) and that was consistently responsive to the needs of the poor. The completed project was also successfully transferred to COMPESA, the state-level maintenance organization, which demonstrated coordination between different organizations. Finally, most of Project R3 (i.e., 95 percent) was completed within a single gubernatorial term, demonstrating continuity in political support for the project. All combined, these characteristics indicate a stable alignment of interests around this project.

The condominial sewer project itself captivated local practitioners and residents. Knowledgeable condominial sewer employees of the municipal and state implementing organizations unanimously identified Project R3 as among the best performing projects in Recife. Residents in the project area overwhelmingly reported high levels of satisfaction with their condominial sewer system from the start of project operation to the time of my fieldwork (five years after implementation); residents gave the project high ratings for operability; and residents reported significant improvements to local health and environment which they attributed to the condominial sewer project. Project R3 left plenty of strong traces that I was able to observe and measure in the field, such as the number of homes connected to the project, the presence or absence of graywater and sewage in the street, and the condition of pipes and manhole covers. These traces allowed me to confirm the relative state of performance at a given point in time. The project's performance level was intimately tied to the actions of the actors to which the project was associated: the performance of the residents, the performance of the implementing organization, and the performance of the officials. These complex associations between residents, implementing organizations, officials, and projects are depicted visually in Figure 6-1. From here forward, I will use the term "project coalition" to refer to the network of associations that form around condominial sewer projects.

Project R3's performance index of 71 (out of 100) was the second highest of the seven condominial sewer projects I studied during Recife and Natal's innovation period. Practitioners unanimously rated it as one of the best performing projects in Recife. Project R3 residents were also the poorest of the seven projects studied. This extraordinary outcome is a shining example of how condominial sewers can be used to overcome social exclusion in infrastructure development. Project R3 accomplished exactly what condominial sewerage is supposed to accomplish: extending urban service to segments of the population that are routinely left out of development. How was Project R3 able to achieve this? The project was obviously inspired by the participatory development model (i.e., which posits that community participation causes better project outcomes), but the participation model alone does not adequately explain the outcome of Project R3. The observations of practice that I have presented clearly demonstrate that Project R3's successful outcome was the effect of a strong and stable project coalition, not the effect of project participation alone. A project coalition-based account recognizes the existence of networks that form around infrastructure projects and takes account of the following: 1) people participate outside the realm of formally designed participation programs; 2) different forms of collective action impact project outcomes differently; and 3) project outcome is a function not only of program design, but of the conditions of implementation in specific times and places. The next project adds additional insights to this understanding of project coalitions.

Project R2

When I arrived in Recife to begin my fieldwork, staff members of the municipal Urban Cleanup Agency (EMLURB) first took me to the Project R2 neighborhood to show me what they characterized as COMPESA's failure.

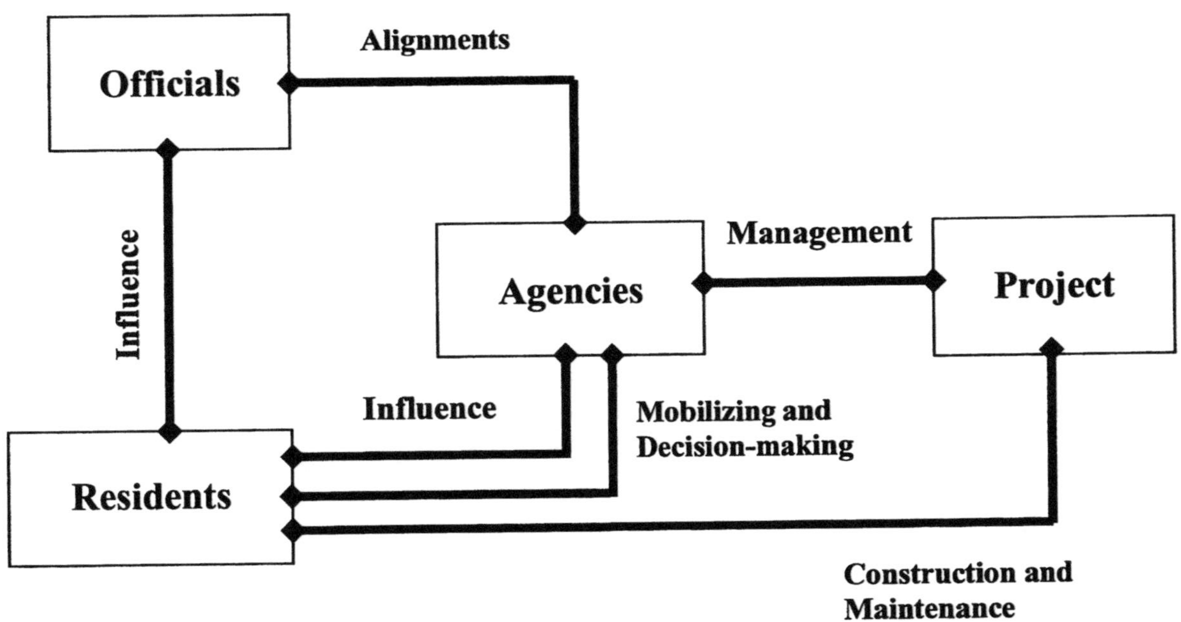

Figure 6-1. Illustration of a project coalition—the network of associations among the actors involved in condominial sewer projects.

A condominial sewer project had been completed there several years earlier, but a conflict was still going on between the city and state organizations involved in water and sanitation projects. The basic issues were bad project performance and project abandonment by COMPESA. Condominial sewer Project R2 had been planned, designed, and installed by the municipal Urban Planning Agency (URB) between 1987 and 1992 in a low-income neighborhood as part of the City's *Projeto Grande Recife* program. The project included condominial sewers (installed in backyards, front yards, sidewalks, pathways, and open areas), treatment of the collected sewage in a community septic tank, and final discharge by pumping to a nearby storm drain.

Project R2 was implemented over the course of several mayoral election cycles. The project had been planned and funded by URB in 1987, then designed in 1988 and re-designed in 1991 by a local engineering consultant hired by URB. The project was subsequently modified again by COMPESA through the same local engineering consultant, constructed by an URB contractor in 1992, accepted and maintained by COMPESA in 1992, and subsequently abandoned by COMPESA about a year later. The EMLURB officials who guided me through the project area were concerned about COMPESA's abandonment of the project and were assessing the project for potential intervention. Surprisingly, Project R2 residents were still receiving monthly sewer bills because their sewer connections still counted as connections even though the majority of the connections were unusable and COMPESA had abandoned its maintenance responsibility for the project. The newly elected Mayor Jarbas Vasconselos had given EMLURB the responsibility of providing backup maintenance on condominial sewer projects that had been abandoned or simply not accepted by COMPESA, while at the same time the mayor was negotiating a binding (by law) agreement with COMPESA on the division of maintenance responsibilities between state agency and municipal agencies.

My first visit to the Project R2 area was alarming. EMLURB personnel and I had to step over and around raw sewage and graywater running through open-air ditches (*valas negras*) in most of the walking lanes and pathways that connected the neighborhood. I observed water supply standpipes and sewer manhole covers that indicated the presence of water and sanitation service, but the condition of these systems was deplorable. Photos 6-2 and 6-3 depict typical scenes of the neighborhood at the time of the fieldwork.

See photo 6-2 in photospread at the end of this chapter.

Project R2 was located in an unplanned, high-density area surrounded by other neighborhoods that were less dense, more urbanized, and higher income. The surrounding neighborhoods had septic tanks, condominial sewer systems, drainage systems, pavement, and normalized housing lots (all installed in the early 1980s), but Project R2 had been left out of these improvements. Like much of Recife, the Project R2 area was very poorly drained and many of the homes were subject to flooding whenever it rained, which created life-threatening conditions because of the ubiquitous presence of raw sewage and the complete lack of any drainage system.

See photo 6-3 in photospread at the end of this chapter.

Urban services were provided sporadically within the R2 project area, with the perimeter having pavement, drainage, electricity, sewers, water supply, and telephone services and the interior having far more limited access to electricity, sewers (barely functioning), water supply (some by outdoor pipe only), and outdoor bathrooms. The streets on the perimeter of the project area were paved and wide enough for access by maintenance trucks, but the interior of the project area had no streets (only unpaved lanes and pathways). Despite the lack of urban services and the appalling sanitation conditions, the Project R2 area still did not have the ubiquitous trash, roaming animals, or substandard housing that were characteristic of Recife's *favelas*; and the average income of the area was low income, not poor. Nevertheless, even though the Project R2 area was technically not a favela, its sanitation conditions had tremendously negative impacts on the lives of residents. Several of the residents I interviewed had been stricken by yellow fever, dengue fever, malaria, chronic diarrhea, dysentery, worms, and other sanitation-related diseases that were more commonly found in poor rural areas and tropical rainforests than in a capital city.

Residents in the Project R2 project area had no informal ties or patron-client relations with state or local officials, but the community's relationship with COMPESA and City agencies could be described as paternalistic. Residents of the adjacent neighborhood were organized into a neighborhood association (*Conselho dos Moradores or Associação dos Moradores*) that was led by a formally elected president. The Project R2 neighborhood was part of this adjacent neighborhood association, whose president also represented the residents of the Project R2 project area. There were two community leaders within the Project R2 area and one community organization (i.e., the Council of Mothers, or *Conselho das Mães*). Residents had not mobilized themselves prior to the project and they did not seek active involvement in the project during implementation. Statements by residents revealed that many of them had become apathetic because of the failure of previous projects in their neighborhood. Previously, URB had installed onsite septic tanks in the Project R2 area under the Recife Program, but these did not function because of the high water table (as high as 1 meter below the ground in some areas). The condominial sewer project came later (under the Grand Recife Program) after the onsite septic tanks had proved to be unsuccessful and with the benefit of the lessons learned from this early attempt to provide sanitation service to the area.

Project R2 suffered from multiple implementation issues including a lack of basic topographic information, delays, and a series of disputable engineering decisions. Topographic information for the area was lacking, and the original scope of work did not include surveying because, according to informants, URB considered this to be a low-cost, basic project and therefore costs had to remain low. The design engineer conducted a rough field survey (unpaid) because he felt it was necessary due to the flatness of the area; he reported that the distances were short and it was difficult to visualize the slopes due to the high density and close proximity of the houses. During the four-year delay between the design and construction of Project R2, URB had difficulties acquiring the privately owned land on which the original pump station and treatment plant were to be sited, so these facilities were relocated. Moreover, COMPESA mandated modifications to the original design, including putting the pump station underground, eliminating the screens and grit chamber (which would have protected the pumps but were considered high-maintenance items), and changing from PVC to clay pipe materials (which were cheaper but more difficult to install in flat areas with a high water table). After design there were more years of delay before the project was built, and unknown additional changes were made in the field during construction.

The original scope of work did not include resident participation or any kind of coordination with the community. At that time, URB's implementation approach did not fully embrace participation by beneficiaries. Residents were not asked to sign, authorize, or accept the system, and they were not involved in decisions such as selecting the level of service, the tariff level, or the system layout. Project staff reported that residents were only spoken to in a limited way every now and then regarding the location and layout of the system in their neighborhood and private lots. Only twice during project implementation did COMPESA and URB conduct house-by-house conversations with residents (in the morning) and a project meeting with residents and the neighborhood president (in the afternoon). The majority of residents said they could not afford to build their house connections to the condominial sewer. Very few of the residents I interviewed knew about project meetings or participation, and most reported that they were not involved in the project. A project inauguration ceremony was held six months after project completion. Less than a dozen residents attended because so few residents had connected to the sewer system by that time. COMPESA abandoned the project soon afterwards. Residents complained about bad project performance to the neighborhood association president in several community meetings, and they mobilized to complain to the City as well. The neighborhood association president estimated that he complained verbally, in person, and in writing about ten times to URB and COMPESA; he also gathered signatures from residents to accompany his written complaints, but the complaints were never answered. At the time of my fieldwork, only 46 percent of the sampled residents in the Project R2 area were connected to the condominial sewer system.

Project R2 residents had little to no involvement in project mobilizing and decision-making; however, community contributions to construction and maintenance were the highest of any of the seven projects I studied. Even though this project had no formal participation program, residents had constructed their own connections, and because of the system's poor performance residents had logged many hours maintaining both the private and public parts of the system (for example, see Photo 6-4). Project R2 achieved a score of only 12 on the sewer performance index, reflecting nearly complete failure. This low score indicates that few, if any, of the twenty-seven performance measures that made up the index were realized to a satisfactory level. All of the practitioners and residents I spoke to agreed that Project R2 was a failed project in terms of performance; and practitioners unanimously rated it as one of the worst performing condominial sewer projects in Recife. Unlike the poor residents of Project R3 described previously, the low-income residents of Project R2 were not able to exert much influence over the course of events in their neighborhood. The R2 area was very small, containing a 1995 population of only 705 people, and the residents were not well organized compared to other neighborhoods in Recife. The residents had not mobilized autonomously prior to the project and did not involve themselves actively in the project during implementation. Notwithstanding this fact, one wonders whether an early outpouring of interest by residents could have increased the accountability of the implementing agencies involved and resulted in a better performing project. But in this case, statements from the residents reveal that many of them had become apathetic because of the failure of previous projects in their neighborhood.

In addition, Project R2 did not benefit from a stable alignment of interests that could have ensured a smoother and less disjointed implementation process. There was no continuity of support by the multiple elected officials and implementing organizations involved in this project over the six-year implementation period. The implementing organizations, URB and COMPESA, were not supportive of condominial sewer technology at the time and did not coordinate their efforts to ensure accountability in the engineering and construction of this project. In sum, the project coalition for Project R2 was too weak and unstable todeliver a viable project, despite very high levels of contributions by residents toward project construction and maintenance. Only one of the linkages in Figure 6-1 that holds the project coalition together was present in Project R2; therefore the project not only failed to perform as desired, its very existence was in jeopardy.

See photo 6-4 in photospread at the end of this chapter.

The Remaining Projects

Similar ethnographic methodology (i.e., holistic description based on fieldwork, observations, and interviews) was applied to the remaining five projects to reveal their actors, relationships, and outcomes. These characteristics, loosely summarized in Tables 6-1 and 6-2 in terms of alignments, influences, participation, and performance, allow me to make two additional points. First, the impact of community participation on project outcome was somewhat ambiguous. Most of the selected projects performed well with only low to mid levels of participation in mobilizing and decision-making, and projects performed well no matter what level of participation in construction and maintenance was achieved. Figures 6-2 and 6-3 show this pattern graphically.[3] Surprisingly, participation in construction and maintenance was not positively associated with performance, contradicting the outcome presumed by the community participation model On the other hand, participation in mobilizing and decisions was positively associated with performance, which supports the community participation model.

Second, there were important differences between Recife and Natal that impacted project outcome. For the projects in Recife, good performance was associated with an alignment of interests, high community influence, and at least mid-level participation in mobilizing and decision-making. Community influence was a critical element in Recife, whose innovation period was characterized by conflict over condominial sewer technology. For the projects in Natal, good performance was associated with an alignment of interests and a consistent participation program applied across all projects. Community influence was not an important element in the formation of project coalitions during Natal's innovation period. Only one of the four studied project communities in Natal was well-organized during project implementation and only one had any notable relationships with officials (Project N4). Furthermore, the neighborhood associations and presidents of all four project communities were inactive at the time of the fieldwork, indicating little perceived need to maintain ongoing pressure and influence in Natal. Residents in all of the project communities did respond very well to CAERN's participation program, however. CAERN's centralized condominial sewer development approach and its use of sewer basins as the basic project unit reduced the importance of community influence in Natal's context. Consequently, good performance was achieved in communities with low influence across a range of income levels.

Project coalitions formed more readily and lasted longer in Natal than in Recife during the period studied. Recife's ad hoc approach to sanitation development produced short-lived project coalitions. This explains why there were fewer good performing projects in Recife overall, and why all three factors were needed to achieve the few instances of good performance that did emerge. Natal, on the other hand, had the benefit of a decade of alignments between elected officials and CAERN, as well as the professional commitment of CAERN staff to condominial sewer technology and a participation approach. With few exceptions, most condominial sewer projects implemented in Natal performed reasonably well no matter what level of community influence was achieved.

The inclusion of residents in project mobilizing and project decisions strengthened the project coalition. However, condominial sewer performance did not necessarily improve when residents focused all their efforts on making contributions to project construction and maintenance because many of the residents were not trained and were unfamiliar with sewer systems. It is not surprising that actions by the organization(s) responsible for implementing sanitation projects were directly tied to project outcomes. In urban settings with an established sanitation organization, the actions of that organization to implement and

Table 6-1. Summary of project characteristics in terms of alignment and influence.[a]

Case	Alignment of Interests					Community Influence				
	Agency Support for the Condominial Approach	Agency Responsiveness to Popular Needs for Sanitation	Project Completion within a Continuous Regime	Coordination between Different Implementing Agencies	Overall Alignments	Average Income Level of the Project Area[b]	Population Size of the Project Area	Degree of Organization of the Project Area	Relationships with Officials	Overall Influence
R1	✓	✓	✓	✓	Stable	✓	1327	✓	✓	High
R2					Unstable		705			Low
R3	✓	✓	✓	✓	Stable		6340	✓	✓	High
N1	✓	✓	✓	✓	Stable	✓	1789			Low
N2	✓	✓		✓	Stable		3535			Low
N3	✓	✓		✓	Stable		3663			Low
N4	✓	✓	✓	✓	Stable	✓	668	✓	✓	High

a. Checkmarks indicate the consistent presence of a factor compared to other projects. No checkmark indicates that the factor was not significantly present. Overall characteristics are suggested by summing the number of checkmarks.

b. I used average household income in each project area as a proxy measure of socio-economic level.[4]

Source: All of the source data used to develop this table is from fieldwork I conducted at the end of the innovation period in Recife and Natal (1994-1995). The selected projects were implemented between 1986 and 1992. Methods of data gathering included interviews with random samples of residents, interviews with community leaders, interviews with engineering and maintenance employees, project area censuses, direct observations, participant observations, project inspections, project area transect walks, and focus groups. See Nance (2004) for the raw data on each project.

Table 6-2. Summary of project characteristics in terms of participation and performance.[a]

Case	Participation						Performance		
	Mobilizing	Decisions	Construction	Maintenance	Index of Participation in M&D	Index of Participation in C&M	Operability	Beneficial Impacts	Index of Performance
R1	✓	✓		✓	54	46	✓	✓✓	67
R2			✓✓	✓✓	4	86			12
R3	✓✓		✓	✓✓	54	63	✓	✓✓	71
N1	✓		✓	✓	38	60	✓	✓✓	68
N2	✓		✓✓	✓	41	59	✓	✓✓	66
N3	✓		✓✓	✓	34	60	✓	✓	55
N4	✓✓		✓✓	✓✓	48	83	✓	✓✓	72

a. Numbers indicate index scores on an ordinal scale from 0 to 100. Single checkmarks indicate a medium or average level of a factor compared to other projects; double checkmarks indicate a substantially higher level of a factor compared to other projects. No checkmark indicates that the factor was not present at an appreciable level. Overall characteristics are suggested by summing the number of checkmarks.

Source: All of the source data and index scores used to develop this table are from fieldwork I conducted at the end of the innovation period in Recife and Natal (1994-1995). The selected projects were implemented between 1986 and 1992. Methods of data gathering included interviews with random samples of residents, interviews with community leaders, interviews with engineering and maintenance employees, project area censuses, direct observations, participant observations, project inspections, neighborhood transect walks, and focus groups. See Nance (2004) for the raw data on each project.

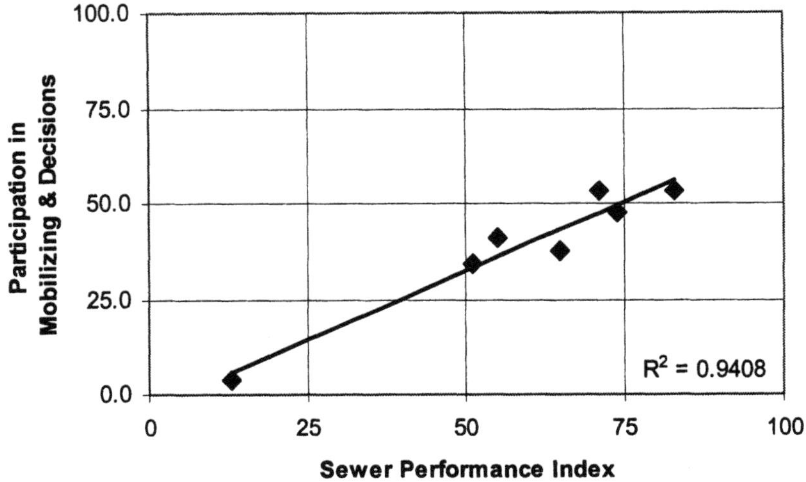

Figure 6-2. Direct comparison of participation in mobilizing and decision-making with the project performance index for seven condominial sewer projects in Natal and Recife.

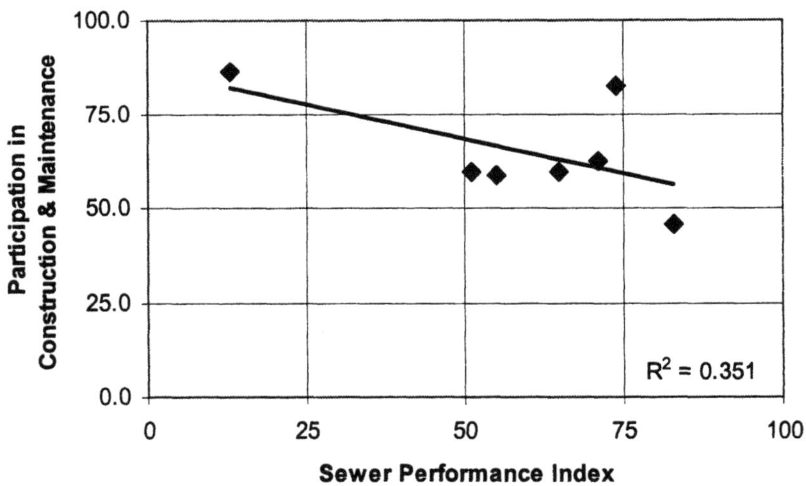

Figure 6-3. Direct comparison of participation in construction and maintenance with the project performance index for seven condominial sewer projects in Natal and Recife.

maintain the sewer system directly affected system performance more than actions by any other actor. When the sanitation organization performed better, the project performed better. In some cases, the actions of elected officials and residents enabled, supported, and supplemented the actions of the implementing organization; in other cases these actors undermined the implementing organization or otherwise affected the project directly.

When politicians, sanitation organizations, and residents formed a strong, cohesive project coalition with staying power, good project performance was more likely. Residents' participation in mobilizing and their involvement in project decisions provided local knowledge and clear expressions of local needs to the sanitation organization, thus enabling the organization to perform better during project implementation. However, while the participation of residents during the project implementation period may have facilitated the installation of a project, it was not enough to sustain good performance in the long term. This is why all of the actors in the project coalition remain important throughout the life of the project. For example, residents in Recife had to constantly exert influence or pressure on the implementing organization and on elected officials to maintain a coalition of support for the project and to ensure continued sewer service. To the extent that the interests of residents were taken into account, project coalitions were made stronger, more durable, and better able to succeed in producing a successful project. In general, a durable project coalition had a better chance of delivering and sustaining a project than a weak, short-lived coalition.

Project Coalitions: An Ethnographic View of Development

The notion of a project coalition was derived inductively from my ethnographies of projects that were constructed during the periods of innovation in Natal and Recife. Project coalitions can be considered an extension of Korten's (1980) conception of "fit" which he used to describe the conditions for implementing successful development projects.[5] Korten proposed that the organization, the beneficiaries, and the project are tightly linked, and that a successful implementation occurred when all three parameters achieved a high degree of "fit." To achieve fit, Korten hypothesized that the following must occur: a project must match the perceived needs of beneficiaries, beneficiaries must have effective ways of expressing their needs to the appropriate implementing organization, the organization must be responsive to these needs in its decision-making and, finally, the implementing organization must have the capacity to effectively carry out its work.

The idea of a project coalition extends Korten's conception of fit by adding a political dimension and by providing further observations about the nature of causality. The trio of parameters that make up Korten's conception are the *organization*, the *beneficiaries*, and the *project*. The project coalition, however, is comprised of the *organization*, the *community*, the *project*, and the *elected official*. The data from Recife and Natal suggest that when the interests of elected officials and implementing agencies were aligned in support of condominial sewer projects (or at least not in opposition), stronger project coalitions were able to form and project success was more likely. Project residents also were important actors in the coalition, as they strengthened project coalitions by participating in the project and by exerting influence on officials and organizations. When alignments were stable over a long period, as they were in Natal, community influence was not particularly important. But when alignments were constantly shifting, as they were in Recife, strong community influence was needed in order to keep project coalitions from falling apart.

Perhaps the most important resemblance between fit and project coalitions is the nature of the relationships between the actors. Korten used double-pointed arrows to represent interdependent relationships between and among the actors. By doing this, Korten was saying that the nature of the causality was not the linear type of causality usually represented by a vector (i.e., a line representing force with an arrow on one end indicating the direction of causality). Rather, the nature of causality was mutually intersubjective, recognizing that, for example, implementing organizations do not exist without projects and projects do not exist without organizations, and so forth. The existence or performance of each is stabilized by their interactivity; one does not really stand alone, disconnected. The network of actors in a project coalition is similarly held together by negotiated associations through which actors engage with each other in the collective creation of a project. At first the new project is a figment, a design, a shared idea held in common among actors. As the associations become more durable, the project becomes more real, more solid, its existence more secure. Once physically constructed, the engineers, officials, residents, and other human actors encounter the project, for the first time, on its own terms. They literally stand back and wait for the project to "act," hence its new status as an actor.[6] Project creation is not, therefore, the result of a simple cause-and-effect link from program design to outcome; rather, it is a series of interactions and evolving associations that intertwine the social and the material.[7]

Not only do project coalitions provide a robust explanation for variations in the observed performance of projects during Natal and Recife's innovation period, project coalition theory is a post-structural extension of Korten's early theory of *fit*, which he used to understand development outcomes. Advancements in post-structural thought and actor-network theory can be used to perform a deeper analysis of fit. Instead of an *a priori* designation of the actors and an *a priori* classification of which type of program design is universally important for success, project coalition theory necessitates the identification of which actors are in play for a particular project and the evolving nature of their associations for a particular time period, recognizing that both the set of actors and the nature of the associations are subject to transformation throughout the life of a project.

Korten's fit theory identifies a generalized set of actors and recommends desired types of associations that produce successful outcomes, but in practice the set of actors can change, and their associations may exhibit a wider range of possible characteristics that change and evolve over time. It is not enough to declare upfront that a particular style of association among a fixed set of actors (e.g., the singular one characterized by fit theory) leads to good performance. One must examine how the conditions of the project coalition in a specific time and place are associated with a particular project outcome. For example, in tracing the network of associations formed among the various actors for the seven selected projects, I found the following: 1) interests between government officials and implementing agencies were in various states of alignment; 2) the influence exerted by project area residents on officials and agency staff varied; 3) there was a range of process inputs by the community (via participation in mobilizing and project decision-making); 4) there was a range of material contributions by the community (via participation in project construction and maintenance); 5) different agencies took various actions to implement projects; and 6) projects took a variety of forms and qualities.

The nature of the associations among actors for the seven selected projects, which was previously introduced in Tables 6-1 and 6-2, is now illustrated visually in Figures 6-4 through 6-8 for three different categories of project outcome: bad, good, and best. None of the outcome measures are absolute; all are relative for the seven selected projects based on a performance index.[8] In all of these figures, a solid black line indicates a relatively strong and stable association during the project implementation period; and a dotted gray line indicates a relatively weak and short-lived linkage. For example, community influence is the ability of residents to persuade project officials and agency staff to take the community's interests into account, and likewise the desire of officials and agencies to be so persuaded. If community influence was particularly strong during the time period observed, this is visually presented in the figures as a solid black line with a two-way arrow. If community influence was ineffective or non-existent during a project, this is visually presented as a dotted gray line with a two-way arrow. Likewise, an alignment of interests exists when officials and implementing agencies each have an interest in working as allies in support of a particular project. If interests were aligned between these actors, this is visually presented as a solid black line with a two-way arrow. If an alignment of interests was unstable or did not exist for a particular project, this is visually presented as a dotted gray line with a two-way arrow. In contrast to the assumed universality of the concept of fit, the project coalitions in Figures 6-4 to 6-8 reflect specific projects in specific times and places and cannot be generalized to other projects, times, or places. Furthermore, in contrast to the static set of associations recognized by the concept of fit, these figures show that different types of project coalitions representing different qualities of associations between actors can each result in a good outcome.

Figure 6-4 shows the project coalition for two of the best performing projects studied as measured by the performance index (R3 and N4). In both of these projects, officials and agencies were aligned in their support for the project, the community successfully exerted influence on officials and agencies to maintain support for their project and to ensure continued service, the community was engaged in all forms of project participation (including mobilizing, decision-

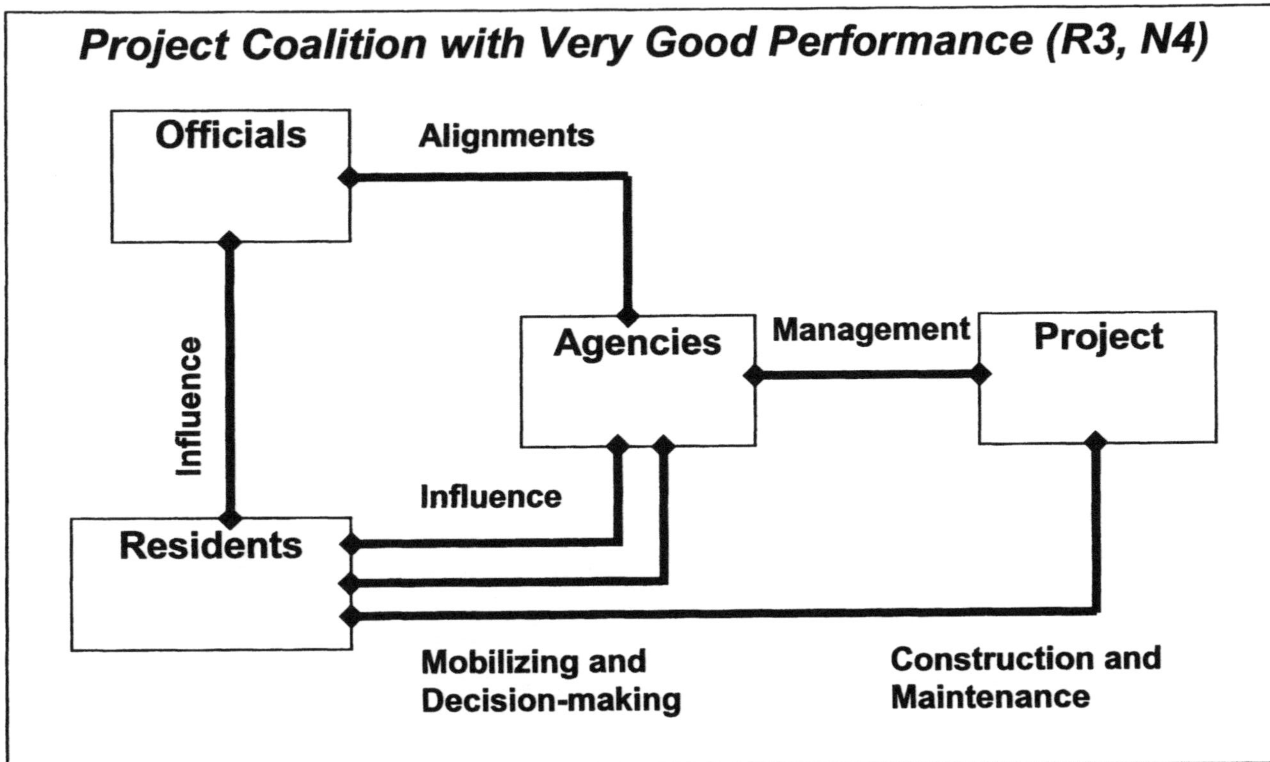

Figure 6-4. Project coalition for two projects with very good performance (R3 and N4).

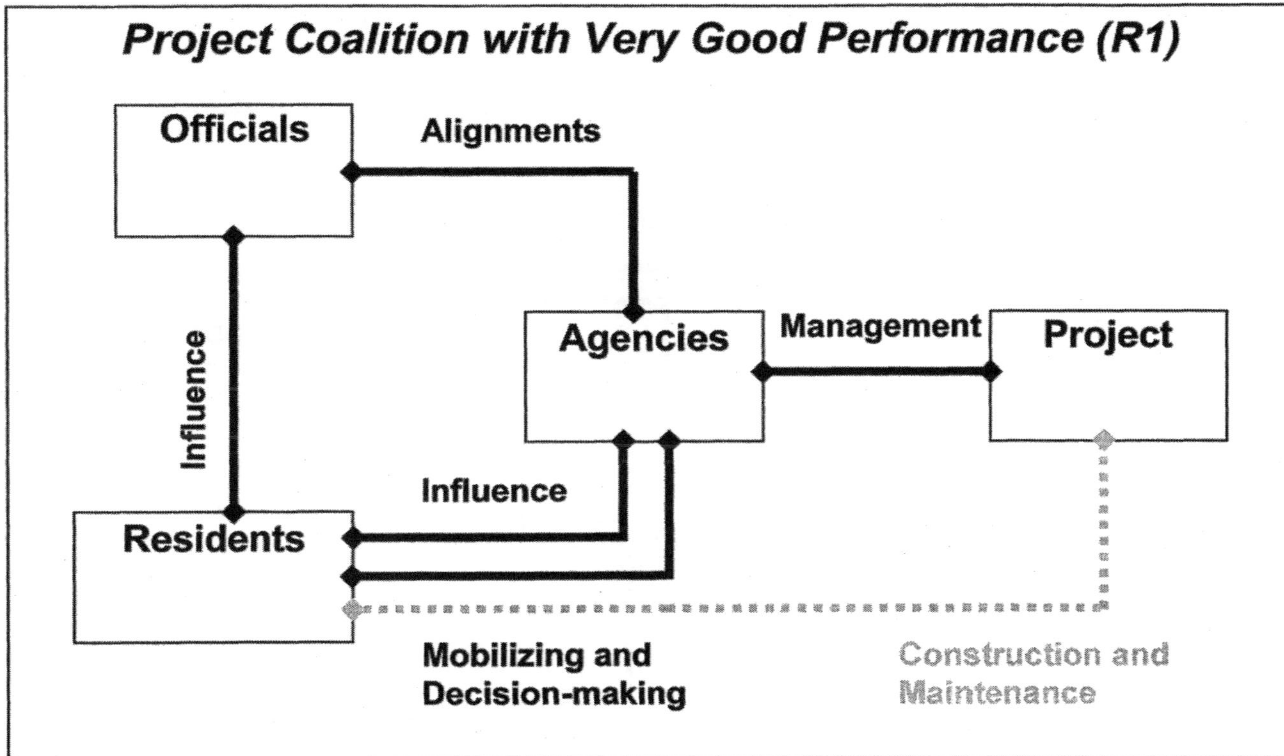

Figure 6-5. Project coalition for a project with very good performance (R1).

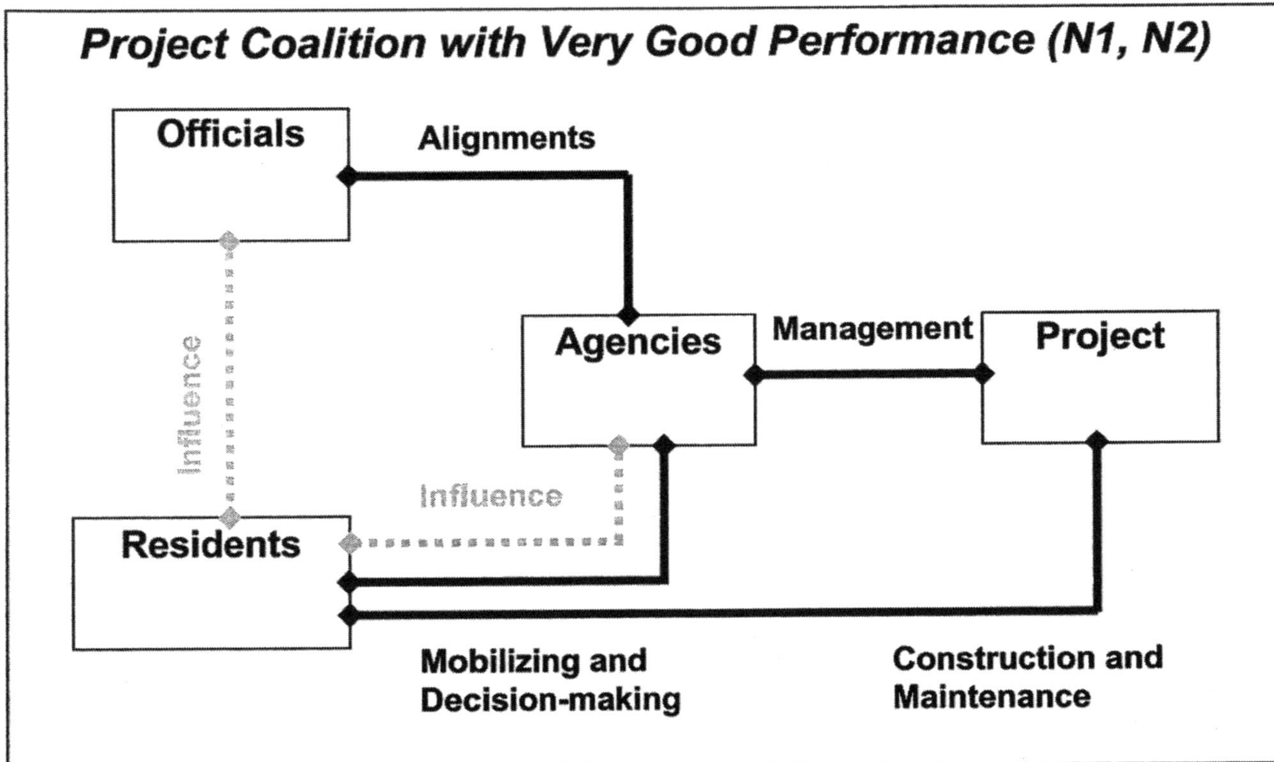

Figure 6-6. Project coalition for two projects with very good performance (N1 and N2).

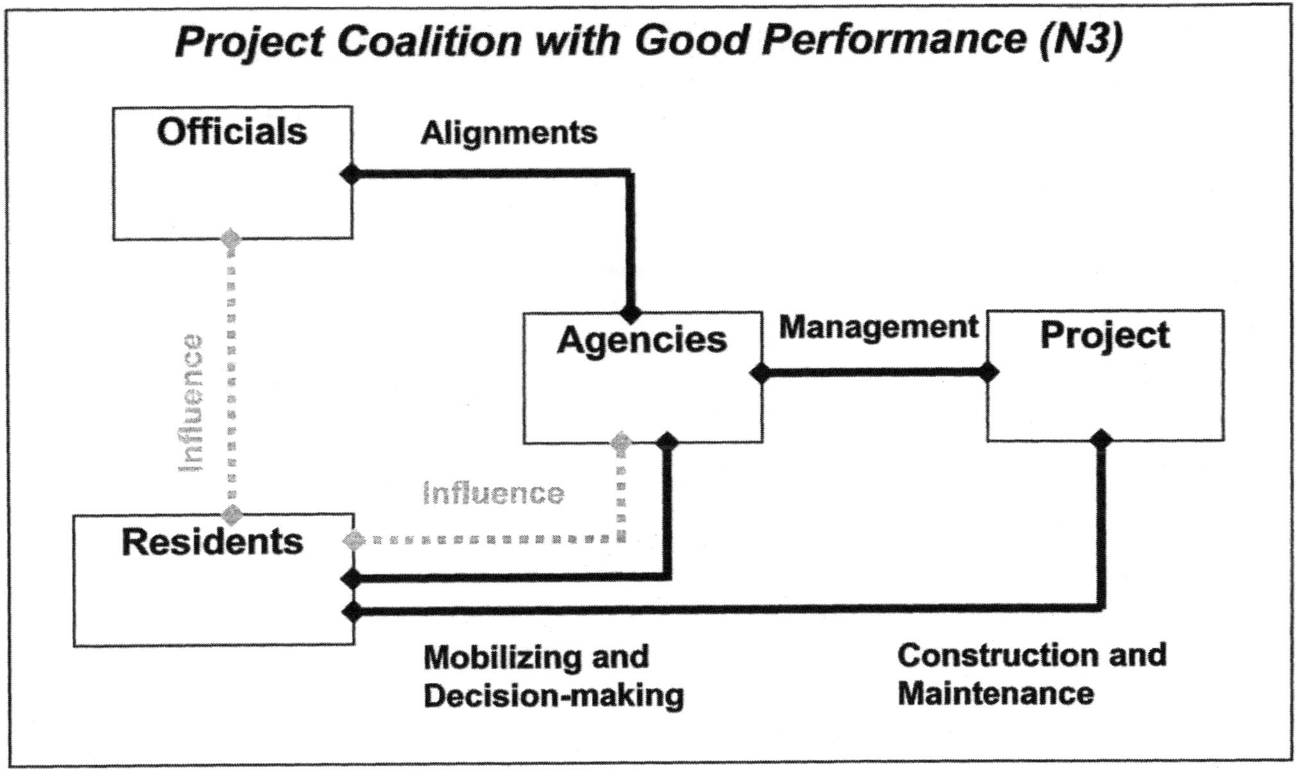

Figure 6-7. Project coalition for a project with good performance (N3).

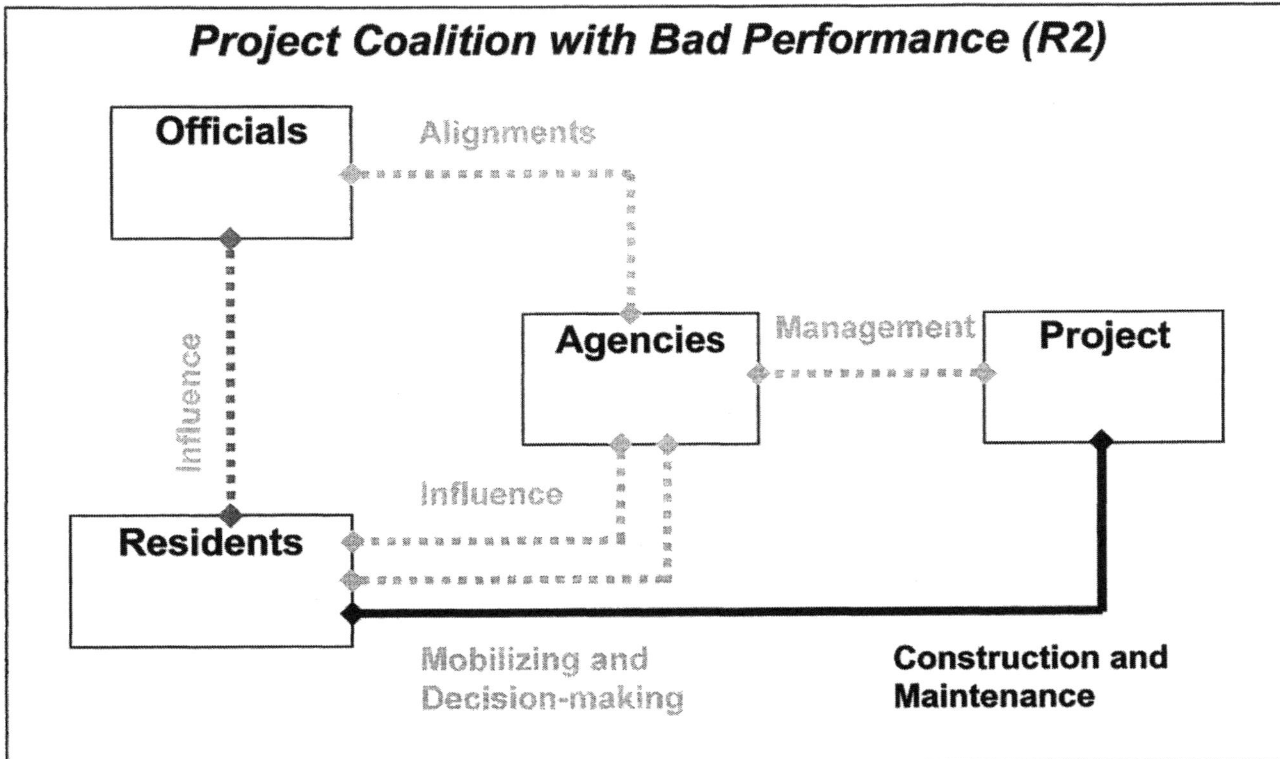

Figure 6-8. Project coalition for a project with bad performance (R2).

making, construction, and maintenance), and the agency completed all of the necessary actions required to implement the project. These two successful projects were characterized by strong and stable associations among all of the actors. The findings in Figure 6-4 demonstrate that outcome was not only associated with participation; it was associated with a strong and stable project coalition that could endure through the election cycles and funding changes that took place during the innovation period in both Recife and Natal.

Figure 6-5 presents a similar finding for another very successful project in Recife (R1). In this instance, participation in construction and maintenance activities was extremely low to non-existent. Nevertheless, the lack of this form of participation had no negative impact on project outcome (as measured by the performance index), thus demonstrating that this form of participation was not necessary for success as long as a strong and stable project coalition was able to endure.

During Natal's innovation period, success was also possible without strong levels of community influence, as shown in Figure 6-6 for two highly performing projects (N1 and N2) and in Figure 6-7 for a project with good performance (N3). Residents exerted very little influence on the officials and the implementing agency for these three projects. However, residents were directly involved in both forms of agency-designed project participation, officials and the implementing organization were aligned in their interests around these projects, and the organization carried out its normal implementation duties as expected. Figures 6-6 and 6-7 demonstrate that communities without influence can be part of a successful sanitation project when the project coalition is strong and stable, and that the standard forms of project participation can and do contribute to the strength of the project coalition.

Finally, Figure 6-8 presents the coalition for a project with bad performance in Recife (R2). These residents were highly involved in construction and maintenance activities (the highest of all projects studied), but they were not involved in mobilizing and decision-making. Like the cases in Figures 6-6 and 6-7, these residents exerted little to no influence. But in this case, the officials and the implementing organization were not aligned in their support for this project and the organization abandoned the project approximately one year after its construction. As a result, the project coalition was weak to non-existent, and extreme levels of community participation in construction and maintenance could not replace the essential network of associations needed for a successful outcome.

A key finding of the foregoing analysis is that relationships among the primary actors varied significantly from project to project. Four different types of project coalitions emerged from the seven projects studied, indicating considerable diversity rather than uniformity in the associations necessary to produce good outcomes during Natal's and Recife's innovation period. Although it was not presented in detail here, there was also considerable diversity in which actors were involved in the various projects; for example, some projects were implemented by multiple agencies and others were implemented by only a single agency. Most interesting is that all of the projects studied gave the "effect" of participatory development; that is, each of the seven projects studied achieved mid- or high-level participation in either mobilizing/decision-making participation or construction/maintenance participation. This was expected because all of these condominial sewer projects were inspired by the same community participatory model, and for this reason these projects could be used to "validate" that model in a very rudimentary fashion. But such spurious analysis would miss the point. The more significant finding is that all of the relevant actors and forces—community influence by residents in the communities being served by projects, alignment of interests between officials and implementing organizations, participation in mobilizing and decision-making—were necessary to fully understand why some projects performed better than others.

It was also necessary to break down the concept of participation in order to see which forms of participation were actually associated with good performance. Participation in construction and maintenance was not as significant as participation in mobilizing and decision-making for the projects studied. Nevertheless, the formation and maintenance of a project coalition, not participation, was found to be the most significant set of actions associated with project performance, per se. Strong and stable coalitions were associated with better performance, and weak and short-lived coalitions were associated with bad performance. In discourse, these projects were labeled "participatory" by default (i.e., because they were condominial sewer projects); but in practice, it was only when the actors successfully established a durable project coalition that measurably good project outcomes emerged.

Closing Remarks for Chapter 6

Chapter 6 compared the condominial sewer implementation experiences of Natal and Recife for the purpose of analyzing the important themes that were introduced in chapters 4 and 5. The key actors were defined in each setting, and the nature of the project coalitions that linked the actors was analyzed for specific projects. The analysis revealed the conditions of coalition formation and illustrated what people were inspired to do on behalf of an innovative sanitation technology. The existence and performance of projects was contingent on the strength and stability of coalitions of elected officials, implementing organizations, and communities that emerged in relation to the project. For the times and places studied, condominial sewer project coalitions were strong and stable when interests were aligned, when communities exerted influence, and when communities participated in project mobilizing and decision-making. The notion of actors forming a project coalition aids in understanding why some projects failed to survive and why others flourished, and the comparative analysis of Natal and Recife revealed the conditions in which project coalitions became either strong and stable or weak and short-lived. An actor-oriented account recognized the existence of networks that formed for the purpose of developing a shared object—a condominial sewer project. Moreover, project coalitions explained project performance more accurately than the community participation model of development by taking account of the following: 1) different forms of participation impacted project outcomes differently; 2) people participated outside the realm of government-designed participation programs; and 3) project outcome was a function not only of program design, but of the conditions of implementation in a specific time and place. While projects were inspired by community participation, in practice it was the strength and stability of the project coalition that was associated with actual project performance. By applying ethnographic methodology to sewer projects, I have shown that the web of relations among the actors—the project coalition—is the ethos of condominial sewerage. It is this new ethos that allowed Brazil to address head-on the problem of social exclusion in sanitation services. But one additional analysis is needed to appreciate just how engineers and their allies were able to accomplish this feat on a large scale. This last analysis is taken up in the concluding chapter.

Notes

1. For a complete explanation of the methodology used to measure project performance, see Nance (2004 and 2005) and Nance and Ortolano (2007).

2. From chapter 3, CAERN is the State Water and Sanitation Agency for Natal, COMPESA is the State Water and Sanitation Agency for Recife, URB is the Recife Urban Planning Agency, and EMLURB is the Recife Urban Cleanup Agency (formerly the Recife Public Works Agency, OBRAS).

3. These seven selected projects are not intended to be representative of all projects. They are intended to be indicative of particular circumstances in which success/failure outcomes occurred in specific times and places.

4. According to the Brazil Census Bureau, "indicators related to the familial nucleus may provide a more comprehensive analysis of the socio-economic situation. . . . A relevant indicator, for example, is the income earned together by family members." IBGE, www.ibge.gov.br/english/presidencia/noticias/12062003indic2002.shtm, 3 March 2004, 11–12.

5. Korten, 1980, 495–98.

6. This idea is from Pickering (1995).

7. Latour often uses the term "actants," an elision of "actor" and "agent."

8. The exception is the category of "best" performance. To earn this characterization, projects had to score among the highest on the performance index *and* be unanimously identified as among the best performing projects in their respective city by local practitioners. See Nance (2004, 71; 2005, 490–93) and Nance and Ortolano (2007, 287–89) for more details.

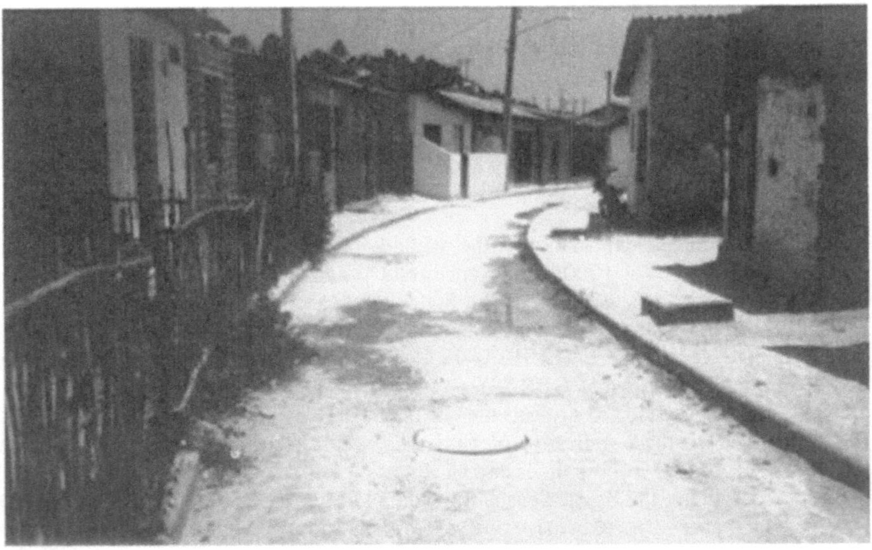

Photo 6-1. Typical street scene for Project R3 as of 1995. (Source: Photograph taken by the author, 1995).

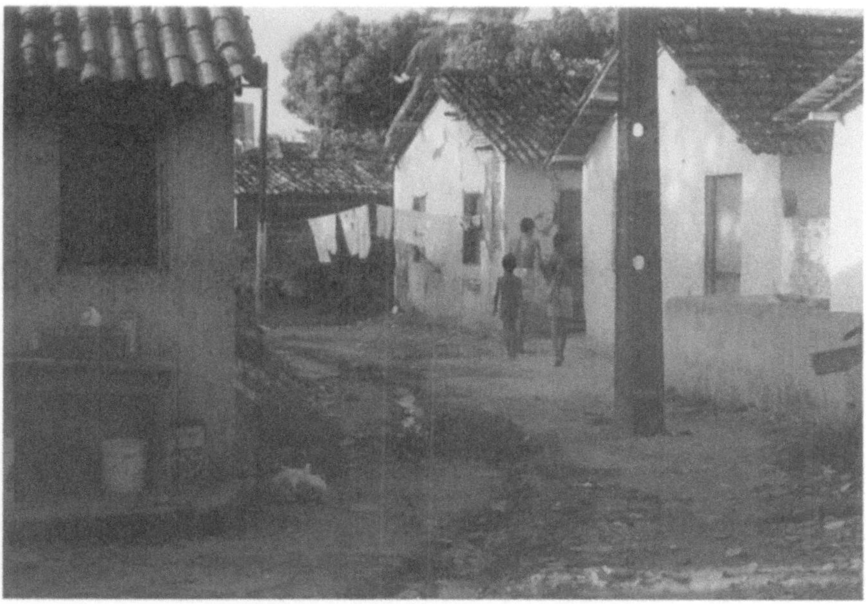

Photo 6-2. Typical street scene for Project R2 as of 1995. Note the open-air sewage ditch (vala negra) running through the main path of the neighborhood. (Source: Photograph taken by the author, 1995).

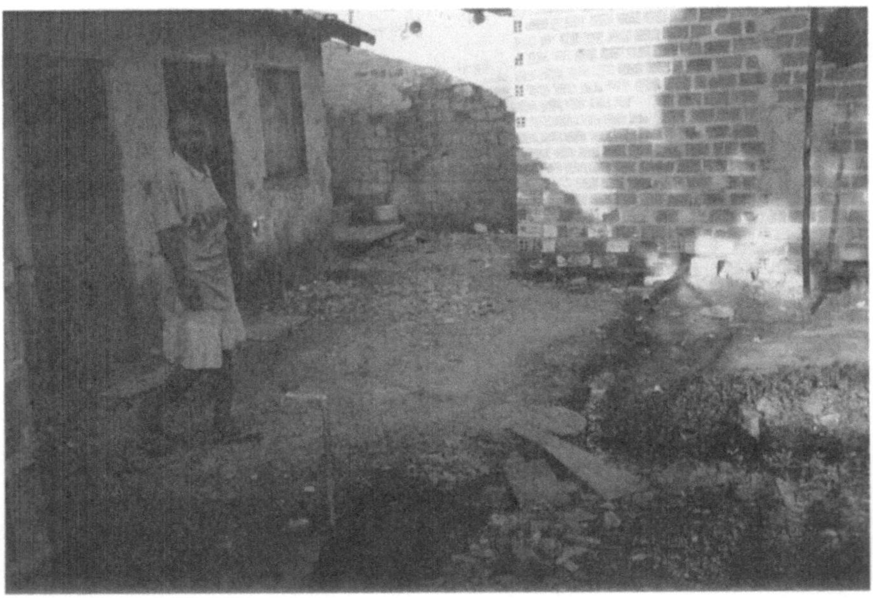

Photo 6-3. Water and sanitation conditions for Project R2 as of 1995. The piped water supply and condominial sewer systems are visible in the photo, but because of the poor performance of the condominial sewer system residents reverted to using an open ditch for the disposal of sewage. (Source: Photograph taken by the author, 1995).

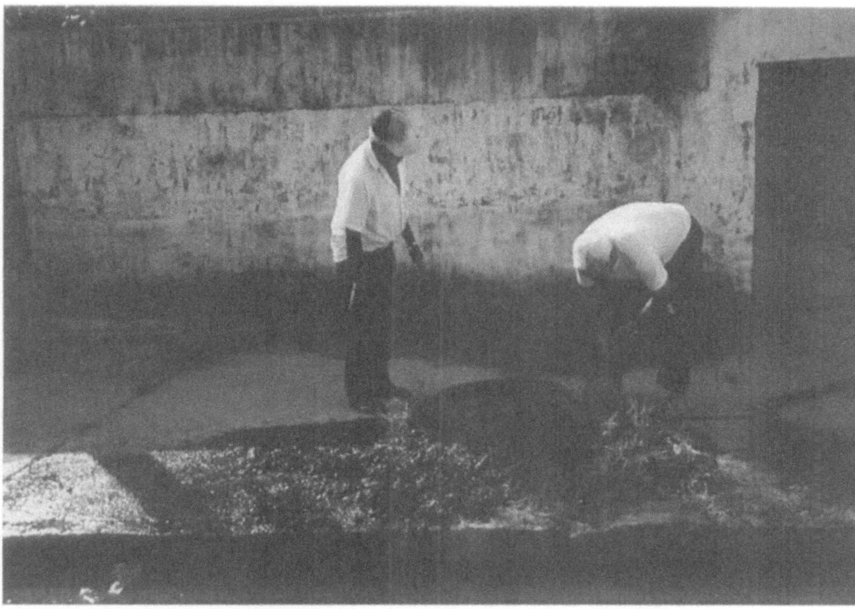

Photo 6-4. Project R2 residents routinely performed maintenance on their condominial sewer system, even on those elements that were located in the sidewalk, a public right-of-way. (Source: Photograph taken by the author, 1995).

Chapter 7
Participatory Sanitation

Researcher: How would you define a condominial sewer system?

Engineer: A simple system that serves one block; that removes sewage from the homes, and that includes participation of the residents. You can have a sewer in the street and it can be a condominial sewer if the people participate and if it is the simplest way to serve all the houses. In Rio de Janeiro, they designed a condominial sewer attached to the walls of favela homes. In Natal, we use backyard condominial sewers because it is the custom, not because this is the definition of a condominial sewer.[1]

Among practitioners of condominial sewer systems in Brazil, this is a typical statement. The notion of participation integrates seamlessly with technical considerations. The statement reflects sensitivity toward local customs and the needs of people who live in a range of conditions. Perhaps most notably, the engineer speaks of systems at the scale of a single block or neighborhood that involve the participation of residents as part of the essence of the system. Statements like these are not typical of most civil engineers or of the engineering discipline as a whole. Within the epistemology of civil engineering, where engineers are "experts," the average citizen is viewed as being unable to offer substantive input to highly technical decisions, and as a consequence citizen participation must "naturally" be limited (within engineering epistemology) to sharing information and educating a public viewed as passive and uninformed. Over time, the conventional infrastructure systems envisioned by civil engineers grew in scale and complexity, in keeping with rising expectations, increasingly rigorous building codes and environmental regulations, and economies of scale. Most civil engineers are engaged in infrastructure solutions that primarily serve the non-poor segments of their populations (regardless of the country) in the name of progress and public safety (measured as industry standards). Indeed, the civil engineering discipline generally constructs its beneficiaries as modern middle-class Westernized citizens. Assumptions about styles of living, such as standard housing types, income levels, access to capital, availability of water, and most generally, the infrastructure needs of a population, reflect a disciplinary bias based on class that, in my view, has contributed to the present predicament of global water and sanitation crisis. No civil engineering department in any major university in the United States has seriously invested in research or teaching about the problems or infrastructure needs of the world's poor, despite the global scale of the problem and the massive potential market. The quote that opened this chapter is therefore unusual not only for who is speaking (a civil engineer), but for the scale of the visualized solution (neighborhoods and households), the implementation approach (participatory), and the intended beneficiaries (the poor). The opening quote could be characterized as a paradigm shift.

A cursory evaluation of the opening quote reveals the key features of this new paradigm. The engineer, a native Brazilian, states that the physical layout of the sewer is not the determining feature; rather, what matters is that it is "a simple solution that serves one block" and that the engineering and construction of the system should not be complex or difficult. Not only is it a low-tech approach, but because the system only serves one block at a time, it is a small-scale project compared to the typical large-scale engineering projects that serve regions and major parts of cities. The physical features of the sewer are based on local conventions rather than industry standards, as evidenced by the statement that "in Natal, we use backyard condominial sewers because it is the custom, not because this is the definition of a condominial sewer." Even the term "condominial" (as in "*esgoto condominial*") does not necessarily provide clear reference to a standard sewer layout or to an expected physical appearance. And the word "sewer" does not necessarily refer to a buried pipe, because "in Rio de Janeiro, they designed a condominial sewer attached to the walls of favela homes." Thus the emphasis is on simple systems that include the participation of residents and that serve all the houses, rather than an emphasis on design standards or physical features. In Brazil, the term *condomínio* was coined to refer to the social arrangement (i.e., user group) that was thought to form among the residents who shared a common sewer collection pipe within a block or group of homes.[2] People's involvement and universal access are therefore important aspects of this new paradigm; perhaps even more important than the physical features of the system. The simple quote that began this chapter reveals the fundamental elements of a new way of thinking about sewerage—simple, small-scale, participatory, and universally accessible. I call this new paradigm "participatory sanitation," in reference to a set of discursive practices about condominial sewers as a social construct, juxtaposed to my use of the term "condominial sewer" to refer to specific projects in the ground that are locally known as *projetos de esgoto condominiais* no matter the details of the physical layout or whether people actually participated.[3]

Collective Constructions

The elements of what I am calling *participatory sanitation*, a variant of a more general discourse on *participatory development*, appear over and over again in written documents and oral statements by condominial sewer practitioners, World Bank staff, project beneficiaries, government officials, and others who speak about and represent condominial sewer projects both within and outside of Brazil. Even though none of these representatives uses the term "participatory sanitation," their discourses about condominial sewers reveal a similar set of ideas and attitudes about the advantages of community participation and appropriate technology. While controversial at first, these ideas have become universally accepted and solidified truths that are now part of a dominant discourse of development that has an overwhelmingly positive view of community participation and appropriate technology. The term "participatory sanitation" is a useful technical term that I will use in tracing the links between condominial sewer practice, discourse about condominial sewers, and discourse about global development.

Dominant Discourses of Development

Since approximately the mid-1980s, the development establishment (e.g., the World Bank, the Department for International Development, the United Nations Development Programme, and so forth) has articulated a discourse of participatory development for extending urban services (especially water and sanitation services) to chronically unserved areas, or, to use the common development jargon, for bringing the poor into development. Most popularly promoted through World Bank Development Reports and United Nations' Millennium Development Goals,[4] this model, in its most generalized form, prescribes at least three key elements for a development program or project to reach the poor: decentralized governance, community participation, and appropriate technology.

The first element, decentralization, imparts the notion that responsibilities and decisions should be devolved to the lowest appropriate level in order to ensure good governance and democratic institutions.[5] Decentralization is thought to ensure voice and accountability between the citizens and the authorities who are responding to the needs of the poor.[6] The following are two examples of how the idea of decentralization has been expressed in widely disseminated statements by the World Bank in the 1990s and 2000s.

> An analysis of World Bank-funded projects demonstrates that a division of responsibilities, provided that there is suitable coordination, leads to better performance and maintenance in the water and sanitation sectors than would be the case in more centralized frameworks. (World Bank, 1994, *World development report 1994: Infrastructure for development*, Washington, DC: Oxford University Press, 75–76)

> Decentralizing delivery responsibilities for public services is prominent on the reform agenda in many developing countries. . . . A key objective, usually linked to the political motivation for decentralization, is to strengthen citizen voice by bringing services and elected politicians closer to the client. . . . Decentralization can be a powerful tool for moving decision-making closer to those affected by it. (World Bank, 2004, *World development report 2004: Making services work for poor people*, Washington, DC: Oxford University Press, 29)

The second element, participation of civil society (i.e., nongovernmental organizations, community-based organizations, households, individual residents, etc.), is also thought to be essential for reaching the poor. It is reasoned that participation by civil society in project implementation and in democratic procedures helps reveal local knowledge and demand, imparts a sense of ownership, increases community capacity, and enhances voice and accountability between users and authorities.[7] Below are two examples of published statements that envision the positive role of participation in development.

> The importance of participation in effective delivery of local public goods is well recognized. . . . A 1985 World Bank review of twenty-five projects (mostly in agriculture and rural development) five to ten years after completion found that participation by beneficiaries and grass-roots institutions was a key factor in those projects' long-term success. (World Bank, 1994, *World development report 1994: Infrastructure for development*, Washington, DC: Oxford University Press, 82)

> How can the role of clients in revealing demand and monitoring providers be strengthened? By increasing poor people's choice and participation in service delivery. (World Bank, 2004, *World development report 2004: Making services work for poor people*, Washington, DC: Oxford University Press, 9)

The third element, the use of appropriate technology, is intended to meet locally perceived needs in ways that are locally acceptable and, especially, locally affordable. The idea is that infrastructure technology should be designed to meet local needs and to be physically, financially, socially, and culturally acceptable.[8] Such technologies, often called low-cost, are no longer regarded as stand-alone solutions; they are part of an overall participatory development approach that includes decentralized organizational arrangements and civil society involvement.[9] Widely available written excerpts that reflect this third element of the participatory development discourse are reproduced below.

> For limited public funding to benefit large numbers, adoption of technical and organizational innovations in low-cost sanitation is necessary. (World Bank, 2004, *World development report 2004: Making services work for poor people*, Washington, DC: Oxford University Press, 89)

> Services must be relevant—filling a perceived need—or there will be little demand for them. (World Bank, 2004, *World development report 2004: Making services work for poor people*, Washington, DC: Oxford University Press, 25)

Statements like those quoted above are quite easy to find, as they have become ubiquitous throughout the development literature produced by a development establishment comprised largely of global development organizations, governmental agencies, and non-governmental humanitarian organizations. It is also not difficult to recognize traces of participatory sanitation within the larger discourse of participatory development, because the paradigm shift that occurred in Brazil's condominial sewerage movement influenced and shaped global discourse on participatory development (as I will demonstrate in later sections of this chapter). The discourse of the condominial sewerage movement was developed in the 1980s and 1990s by Brazilian condominial sewer practitioners, Brazilian engineers, and Brazilian professors; and supplemented by officials from the World Bank and other international development organizations. The 2000s version of participatory sanitation consists of three central ideas: universal access, appropriate technology, and participation. The notion of universal access means that everyone—rich and poor—can be served under the participatory sanitation approach, in contrast to the conventional sanitation approach which has been shown to primarily serve only the wealthiest population segments in Brazil.

Written excerpts of participatory sanitation discourse are readily available in documents produced by condominial sewer practitioners and development agencies. Some examples are reproduced below.

> The two most prominent features of this experience were the achievement of universal access at very low financial cost to the utility company as well as the conscious, consistent way in which the technology was adopted by the utility company, providing service access to a wide socioeconomic spectrum. (José Carlos Melo, "The Experience of Condominial Water and Sewerage Systems in Brazil: Case Studies from Brasília, Salvador, and Parauapebas," World Bank, 2005, 7)

> The 'condominal approach' has two defining features. The first is the use of innovative engineering techniques. . . . The second is the integration of social and engineering work. By involving communities in the construction and maintenance of the condominial networks, further cost reductions are achieved. Moreover, the interaction with the community during the execution of the works provides opportunities to impart hygiene education and to influence water consumption habits in a variety of ways. (Vivien Foster, "Condominial Water and Sewerage Systems: Cost of Implementation of the Model," World Bank, no date, 10)

> By involving residents in project design and implementation, the condominial system can achieve close to 100 percent connection rates. (Gabrielle Watson, "Good Sewers Cheap?: Agency-Customer Interactions in Low-Cost Urban Sanitation in Brazil," World Bank, 1995, 10)

The overall message is that participation and appropriate technology lead to successful projects, where success is measured in terms of universal access. Since the end of the condominial sewer innovation period (i.e., the mid-1990s), the discourses of participatory development and participatory sanitation have been the orthodoxy in water and sanitation development; that is, they have been believed and uncontroversially acted upon by the majority of international development practitioners.

It is interesting to juxtapose Brazil's paradigm shift toward participatory sanitation, which paralleled and influenced the global paradigm shift toward participatory development, against the larger notion of "development" which has been the subject of monumental critique by academic scholars for decades (but especially since the 1980s).[10] Among the leading post-colonial and post-development scholars who have contributed to this critique, Edward Said, James Ferguson, Wolfgang Sachs, and Arturo Escobar have been particularly influential. Said's classic post-structuralist work, *Orientalism* (1979), spelled out the ways in which dominant Western views of the East—solidified into the discourses and practices of colonialism and international development—created, enabled, and perpetuated inequality as part of development. Ferguson's groundbreaking contribution, *The Anti-Politics Machine* (1990), exposed in elegant detail the conceptual apparatus of the dominant development discourse, its constructed version of "less developed countries" as objects of development, and its denial of history and politics in the service of expanding bureaucratic state power. Sachs's highly influential volume, *The Development Dictionary* (1992), argued that the development paradigm, and the web of key concepts that comprise its discourse, has failed on its own terms and that the age of unquestioned development, which was based on "a set of tacit assumptions which reinforce[d] the Occidental world view" (4–5), has come to an end. Escobar's award-winning *Encountering Development* (1995), offered a comprehensive critique of development in which he outlined development practice in historical perspective and revealed how Western development discourse had ordered the world by productively constructing notions of "the poor" and "the underdeveloped" as subjects in need of Western humanity. These authors' brilliant insights about hegemonic power in global development discourse and practice have inspired many and have cultivated the fields of critical development studies, anthropology of development, area studies, and others. It is no longer possible to examine "development" without recognizing that, in Hobart's words, "scientific knowledge as observed in development practice generally represents the superior knowing expert as agent and the people being developed as ignorant passive recipients or objects of this knowledge."[11]

What, then, is the "proper" perspective for an interrogation of condominial sewers (many of which were funded by global development agencies) and participatory sanitation (a discourse now intimately connected to the dominant discourse of participatory development)? Should the Brazilian engineers, practitioners, and local officials, who were themselves enrooted in an oppressive national development structure that had routinely excluded poor people from basic urban services as a matter of course, be viewed as instrumental agents of a dominant development paradigm, should they be viewed as activists trying to change the system from within, or are these categories too simplistic, too fixed, or perhaps even unhelpful? Was the knowledge they created "local," was it imposed by Western development agencies and/or national officials, or were local knowledge and Western scientific knowledge commingled? These questions are significant because they reveal the possibility of epistemological bias in examining local/indigenous innovation in development as this book has attempted (the author is from the United States). Grillo and Stirrat (1997) summarize this predicament nicely:

> The 'Other' is constructed as if, behind an impermeable barrier of epistemology, 'we' can never understand 'them.' . . . [T]here is a real danger of assuming that ignorance is one-sided; that is, it is 'we' who are only and always ignorant. The danger is that indigenous knowledge is seen as complete, accomplished, and hence static and unchanging. Neither side has a monopoly of knowledge or ignorance, neither party is impervious to argument. . . . There often remains, of course, a significant distance between the ideas and practices of development agencies and those of 'local' people. (Grillo and Stirrat, 1997, 24–25)

Grillo and Stirrat (1997) also identify a number of paths out of this potential epistemological trap: a) studies that emphasize local/indigenous conceptions of development and its processes; b) studies that recognize development as multivocal and multi-sited, occurring at project sites, in neighborhoods, in local government offices, capital cities, NGOs, engineering firms, international development agencies, etc.; c) studies that use an "actor-oriented approach that . . . obliges the researcher to acknowledge . . . multiple realities and provides a method for examining the coexistence of [multiple actors and voices]"; and d) studies that problematize development discourse itself.[12] Up to this point in the analysis of condominial sewers and participatory sanitation, I have attempted to carry out the first three of these strategies (to varying degrees). The focus of the first six chapters of the book has been on understanding a locally-defined development solution to a locally-perceived sanitation problem (i.e., *esgoto condominial*) from multiple perspectives (e.g., residents, maintenance technicians, engineers, public officials, contractors, and consultants) and tracing the networks of association among various actors involved in projects located in seven neighborhoods across two cities (i.e., project coalitions). I have saved for this last chapter an explicit analysis of participatory sanitation discourse that will address some of the epistemological issues noted above.

Multiple Discourses of Development

While hegemonic power in global development discourse and practice is a reality, it is not the only reality. Development scholars now recognize the coexistence of multiple discourses of development rather than a single discourse,[13] for example, professional developers, the local people being developed, the national government, and local officials each construct development differently and possess different types of knowledge about development.[14] Even limited observations of local people, practitioners, and officials provide ample evidence of the coexistence of multiple discourses of development. Three such discourses—that of engineers, maintenance technicians, and residents—were illuminated in an analysis of how different stakeholders viewed the performance of condominial sewer projects.[15]

Of the three groups studied, maintenance technicians had the highest degree of within group agreement in their interpretations of condominial sewer performance. Residents also had a high degree of within group agreement about project performance. These findings suggest that maintenance technicians and residents had constructed one aspect of development—project performance—in relatively coherent views that could be called discourses. However, different stakeholder groups scored the same project differently, and maintenance technicians were consistently more critical of condominial sewer performance than engineers and residents. These patterns suggest the coexistence of multiple discourses among stakeholder groups, except that the engineering "group" was not so easily aggregated.

Engineers, especially those directly associated with a development project, are typically the primary group of practitioners involved in project evaluation research. They are often expected to provide "expert" judgments on development indicators (e.g., ratings of performance) and to speak authoritatively about a project from a knowledgeable, scientific perspective. All of the engineers I interviewed for the performance study naturally assumed this role and willingly provided initial judgments of the best and worst performing projects in their respective cities. However, subsequent content analysis of the engineering discourse about performance revealed several surprises. First, the engineers' initial performance judgments were not generally accurate when compared to field measures of project performance. Second, engineers as a group had the lowest degree of agreement in their responses to questions about project performance (compared to the degree of agreement within the maintenance and resident groups). Third, most of the engineers interviewed were unable to rate individual projects on a scale (i.e., in which engineers were asked to rate the performance of specific projects on a 1 to 5 scale), even though the same individuals had confidently provided initial judgments of the best and worst performing projects in response to open-ended interview questions. These findings were consistent in both Natal and Recife, and in all cases the engineers selected were those who had extensive experience with numerous condominial sewer projects in their respective cities, engineers who had served as project manager or project engineer for the specific projects in question, and engineers who were considered local experts on the subject. Given these findings, it is difficult to believe in the notion of a single "engineering discourse." Nevertheless, Brazilian engineers did construct a coherent discourse about condominial sewers (which is analyzed in depth later in this chapter). That discourse was not, however, a completely accurate portrayal of actual project performance. The perspective of the engineers established a discernible gap between participatory sanitation discourse and condominial sewer practice. In the remainder of this chapter I explore this gap.

The Myth of Participatory Sanitation

Using the word "myth" to characterize the participatory sanitation paradigm is not, *de facto*, a derogatory statement. It is intended to be an accurate statement about how the paradigm is actually used, and to contrast the use of *paradigms as myths* to the use of *paradigms as theories* that scientifically "explain" observations. Myth has proved a useful concept for discussing the contradictions of development.[16] During the condominial sewer innovation period in Brazil, the participatory sanitation paradigm was neither an accurate description of on-the-ground project experiences (i.e., it did not function as a scientific theory) nor did it encapsulate the diversity of sanitation discourses that were in existence at any given time and place (i.e., it did not function as a meta-narrative). I argue that it functioned as a myth, roughly synonymous with the notion of metaphor or allegory used in a rhetorical mode and designed to engage interest and motivate action toward creating and maintaining networks of association that were necessary for actual techno-cultural innovation, in this case for solving the sanitation problem.

Janice Perlman made powerful arguments about the role of myth in development in her groundbreaking 1976 book, *The Myth of Marginality*. Perlman examined a wide range of literatures and discourses about poverty and came to the conclusion that they all reflected the same myth (which she called the "myth of marginality"), even though no individual source explicitly expressed that myth *as a myth*. Perlman went on to fully elaborate the myth and then disproved it empirically using evidence from her in-depth case studies. While it is obvious that poverty itself is an objective condition of reality for many people, Perlman successfully showed how mythical conceptions of poverty did not reflect the reality of poor people. In this chapter, I present, similarly, a number of statements, literatures, and texts that are reflective of a mythical conception of participatory sanitation as an idealized image. And, like Perlman, I make reference to situated, project-based evidence that contradicts the paradigm, thus revealing its use as myth rather than as theory. Such an analysis will yield insights into the basis of belief in participatory sanitation specifically and in participatory development in general; and about the crucial role that myth played in efforts to overcome social exclusion in sanitation development. However, I will move beyond simply exposing the myth to offering an explanation for why myth was necessary in the specific historical context of condominial sewer innovation.

Another use of the term "myth" in development studies was contributed by the distinguished international water and sanitation engineer Richard Feachem, who at the beginning of the International Water and Sanitation Decade (1980) published a paper entitled, "Community Participation in Appropriate Water

Supply and Sanitation Technologies: The Mythology for the Decade." In an insightful, even prophetic, analysis, Feachem argued that the "guiding themes" of participatory development in water and sanitation were being applied in an "over-simplified manner and that they divert attention away from the fundamental political and administrative realities that primarily determine the success or failure of rural water and sanitation programmes." The evidence I have presented in this book substantiates Feachem's predictions about the factors that lead to water and sanitation success.

However, my use of the term "myth" deviates somewhat from Perlman's and Feachem's use of the term because I take the position that myth can be used in both constructive and destructive ways. In the case of condominial sewerage I argue that the myth of participatory sanitation was, for the most part, used constructively during the innovation period to open up space to experiment with new ways of overcoming social exclusion in the sanitation sector. I also argue that long-term and large-scale success will necessitate an evolution of the paradigm from myth toward an evidence-based theory of development that encompasses the poor.

Why did some Brazilian civil engineers, such as the one quoted at the beginning of this chapter, suddenly seek to expand sanitation service to the long-unserved segments of their society, which included mostly poor, low-income, and some middle-income residents? These engineers, whom I have called activist engineers (to differentiate them from other engineers who defended the status quo of conventional sanitation), created and disseminated a form of sanitation service that diverged markedly from the conventional forms of service that were standard engineering practice at the time. Given the power of the policies, laws, and standards that protected the civil engineering industry and its conventional sanitation practices, how did these activist engineers manage the difficulties of that transition and what were the consequences? And most importantly, how and why did they go about constructing the paradigm of participatory sanitation? Implicit in this line of questioning is the fundamental argument of the book: that the important innovation was not condominial sewer technology, per se; it was the paradigm of participatory sanitation, which inspired the formation of project coalitions through which experimentation was possible.

This chapter describes the contrasts between how condominial sewers actually performed versus the discourse that was developed for promoting them. This investigation into the basis of belief in and the actual employment of the participatory sanitation paradigm entails an explanation of how order was constructed out of empirical chaos, as well as a description of how alternative readings of project outcomes were eliminated in the process.[17] This line of questioning moves beyond simply identifying the myth in comparison to actual events. It allows me to address a set of questions best laid out by Bruno Latour about what scientists (and engineers) *say* they do versus what is actually *done* in practice. Latour not only identified contradictions between the discursive and the material, he tried to explain the general effect of this contradiction on society. The central question is: If participatory sanitation does not explain reality, then why do engineers use it to explain reality? In the next section, I investigate this question by presenting various versions of the participatory sanitation paradigm as it traveled and evolved from one Brazilian city to the next.

Sewers in Translation: From Natal to Recife to Bahia

After the initial pilot projects, news about participatory sanitation traveled first, followed by actual projects. Activist engineers who represented the emerging condominial sewer technology created oral and written texts (i.e., discourses) to aid the proliferation and expansion of the technology from city to city. The founding spokespeople for condominial sewerage included engineers and social scientists from state water and sanitation companies in Brazil, engineering professors, engineers in private practice in Brazil, and engineers and social scientists from international development agencies (e.g., the World Bank). Founding spokespeople stand out because of their efforts to communicate a consistent narrative to a wide range of people via oral presentations and written publications (several of which are cited herein). Melo, unanimously viewed as Brazil's leading spokesperson on the matter, developed the original condominial sewer narrative in the state of Rio Grande do Norte (as a result of his association with the initial pilot projects in Natal and other towns) in collaboration with spokespeople at CAERN and the Federal University of Rio Grande do Norte (*Universidade Federal do Rio Grande do Norte*, or UFRN). Melo then carried this narrative to his home state of Pernambuco where, through his private engineering practice, he was able to further develop the narrative via condominial sewer projects implemented in several interior towns throughout the Northeast in the early 1980s. In the mid-1980s, he used his position as vice-mayor of Recife (Pernambuco's capital city) to further articulate the narrative, and he continued to guide the emergence of projects in the interior of the state through his subsequent position as State Secretary of Sanitation. With every experience, local narratives proliferated, evolved, converged, and evolved further, but Melo's presence served as a unifying filter through which diverse local experiences merged into a singular paradigmatic narrative.

The initial paradigm of the 1980s emphasized the appropriate technology characteristics of condominial sewer systems (i.e., physical design features that contributed to the system's low-cost), but later versions of the paradigm (ca. the 1990s) emphasized the community participation aspects of the system. Spokespeople presented the initial paradigm at engineering conferences in Brazil and at seminars convened by universities and international development agencies in Brazil and around the world, and they published the initial paradigm in various engineering journals, technical reports, and a doctoral dissertation.[18] By the mid-1990s, Melo had written a book describing the evolving paradigm, in which he portrayed a unified conception of condominial sewerage with particular emphasis on the integral role of participation.[19] At the same time, the World Bank commissioned a comprehensive study of the state of condominial sewerage in seven Brazilian states (mostly in the Northeast).[20] The World Bank also published a special report fully articulating the role of community participation in water and sanitation,[21] and condominial sewerage began to appear as a new alternative in international water and sanitation text books.[22] Statements from Brazilian condominial sewer practitioners in the Northeast expressed the state of the paradigm in action during the mid-1990s (emphases added).[23]

> It's not the physical part that defines a condominial sewer. It's the *involvement of the community* that is 'condominial.' A conventional layout can be a condominial sewer if the people choose the layout and pay the costs. The method of access to the public sewer is the community's decision.
>
> . . . low-cost, shallow depth, and *the community acting as a collective.* If the collective exists, then a condominial sewer exists, whatever the layout.
>
> A more economical alternative that *requires participation and orientation of the users* during implementation.
>
> A rational and logical solution *where people work together* to solve sewage problems. It's the *condomínio.*
>
> Participation—a way of combining the forces of residents and the implementing agency. *Everybody works together* towards the sewer system; the sewer agency does not do everything for the residents.
>
> The *condomínio,* or *collective relationship.* A collective relationship between residents and the implementing agency, and a collective connection between homes and the sewer infrastructure.
>
> If *the residents build it, contract it, or pay the City to build it* then it's a condominial sewer no matter what is the layout. They are also responsible for maintenance.
>
> Condominial sewerage is not a new technology; it's a new relationship between users and government and among *the collectivity of the users* themselves.
>
> Physically, it is defined as a low cost system. Philosophically, it is *defined by the participation of residents* among themselves and by the public agency's actions to stimulate this participation.
>
> A sanitary sewer system that requires *participation of the residents,* and that also has homes interconnected in the backyard, in the front yard, or on the sidewalk. It must have participation because we have to enter the private property of the resident and because one resident can harm others.
>
> A form of sanitary sewerage that brings awareness to the population, *promoting everyone to participate* in the system. This is fundamental: participation.
>
> The major difference is the philosophy. The first thing that's done is to *contact the community and see if they want a condominial sewer.* In conventional sew-

ers the whole project is designed without ever contacting residents. They don't find out about the project until they see construction happening.

It follows the objective of health....To the extent that you are really attending to and serving the people, you are resolving the health problems. . . . The *resolution of sewer problems for the whole community*, and not just for individuals, is a condominial solution.

Like published accounts of the paradigm during the mid-1990s, the above statements from practitioners emphasize the importance of participation (and, to a lesser degree, appropriate design and decentralized organizational arrangements). The participatory sanitation paradigm was consolidating and gaining strength throughout Brazil's Northeast region and beyond (as other states adopted the technology and as the World Bank published the paradigm). No matter whom I asked or what I read, the message was the same. Participatory sanitation was becoming universal and was being translated across great distances.

One route taken in the process of translating the paradigm was from Natal, where condominial sewerage had originated in the early 1980s, to Recife, where the innovation emerged in the mid-1980s, to Bahia in the mid-1990s. Like Recife and Natal, Bahia (also known as Salvador), is a coastal capital city in Brazil's Northeast region that ultimately adopted condominial sewerage. Bahia's adoption, however, occurred after the period of innovation, so (unlike Recife and Natal) Bahia is not considered an early innovator. By the time Bahia was introduced to the participatory sanitation paradigm in 1995, condominial sewer *practice* had actually destabilized in Natal and was on the decline, and in Recife condominial sewer *practice* was being consolidated and was on the rise (after much initial struggle). Circa 1995, a contingent of engineers from Recife traveled to Bahia to offer the participatory sanitation paradigm.[24] The Recife engineers conducted a series of special training seminars in which they taught the paradigm to engineers of Bahia's state water and sanitation company (i.e., *Empresa Baiana de Águas e Saneamento*, or EMBASA). Instead of discussing the actual mixed outcomes of pre-1995 condominial sewer projects available at that time from experiences in Natal, Recife, and other parts of the Northeast, they presented and discussed the newly consolidated paradigm of participatory sanitation, supported by stories from a carefully selected set of successful condominial sewer experiences. EMBASA engineers received a fully articulated version of condominial sewerage by dedicated spokespeople who had constructed a coherent paradigm out of material chaos. The paradigm they presented emphasized two key causal factors which they related to success: appropriate technology (i.e., simple low-cost design) and participation. This was in line with publications emerging from the World Bank at the time. EMBASA adopted the technology and was soon rewarded with World Bank resources to initiate a comprehensive condominial sewer program in Bahia.

Condominial sewers had now been around for fifteen years in Brazil, and it was possible to gather significant evidence of their actual outcomes using on-the-ground data about project performance to date and the conditions in which success and failure had occurred. My in-depth analysis of the projects in Natal and Recife during this timeframe (presented in earlier chapters) is revealing of the contradiction between the paradigm of participatory sanitation (as published and presented) and the range of performance outcomes of condominial sewer projects implemented during the innovation period. All of the projects I studied used appropriate low-cost design features in accordance with the paradigm (therefore this factor was "controlled" in an experimental sense); however, the projects were implemented with varying degrees and different forms of participation, thereby allowing a direct comparison between participation and performance, which serves as a rudimentary examination of the paradigm.[25] My analysis of participation versus performance (in chapter 6) showed that outcomes were not explained by the degree of participation alone, and that participation was not always the most important, necessary, or sufficient factor.

As described at length in earlier chapters, a durable project coalition was the key to successful project performance during the innovation period. The conditions in which durable project coalitions flourished were different in Natal and Recife, depending on the alignment of interests and the exertion of community influence, which were shown to have stronger effects than participation in some cases. My analysis, which selected best and worst cases of project performance during the innovation period in Recife and Natal, found that the actual range of project performance varied significantly and included failures, but that failed projects were either dismissed and ignored or were, at times, erroneously described as successes during the process of paradigm translation. Compounding the denial of failure was a non-critical view of participation that was maintained even in the face of contradictory information.

This was particularly evident in discourse about the two original condominial sewer projects in the neighborhoods of Rocas and Santos Reis, Natal. Operations and maintenance (O&M) staff privately characterized these projects as failures, but engineers (who operated as spokespeople for the technology) publicly characterized these very same projects as successful examples of the participatory sanitation paradigm. For example, the following two sets of statements were presented in 2004 at a national sanitation conference in Brazil by practitioners and officials involved in condominial sewerage. The first statement is by a representative from the National Bank of Brazil, an organization that plays a significant financing role in Brazil's sanitation sector:

> The participatory sanitation model (was) developed in Rio Grande do Norte by (the water and sanitation company) CAERN. . . . A conventional sanitation project was anticipated to serve a maximum of 30 percent of the population. . . . The participatory sanitation pilot project in (the neighborhoods of) Rocas and Santos Reis resulted in a 97 percent connection rate and improved healthfulness of the area. (Source: Mariz, *Tecnologias Alternativas e Integradas para o Saneamento Ambiental*, SANEPAR Congress, Brazil, 2004, slide nos. 23–24; translated by the author)

Observe that this speaker makes selective use of an extremely narrow performance indicator (i.e., the connection rate) to create the perception of widespread success of these two projects. The next set of statements, which refer to the same two condominial sewer projects, was presented by a respected civil engineering professor and consultant who was also one of the "founding fathers" of Brazil's participatory sanitation approach.

> The high connection rate and level of satisfaction of the users in (the neighborhoods of) Rocas and Santos Reis demonstrate the viability and efficiency of the system. However, the agency-community partnership has not been continuously active, resulting in the withdrawal of the parties from the partnership. Among the principal causes of this withdrawal was the lack of resolution of the agency's technical responsibilities, a break in the initial accord (maintenance by residents with agency support), no effort to stimulate the active involvement of the *condomínio*. . . . Despite this evidence, the system has operated satisfactorily for 20 years and the social transformation of the community is perfectly visible. (Source: Neto, *Modelo Condominial de Esgotamento Sanitário: Conceituação nos Aspetos Tecnico e Social*, SANEPAR Congress, Brazil, 2004, slide no. 19; translated by the author)

Note that this statement is internally incongruous. There is a complete disconnect between the evidence provided and the statement's conclusion, again with a bias toward showing a positive view of system performance on the basis of a narrow view of the concept. The speaker reveals fundamental failures in the project coalition (e.g., "withdrawal . . . ," "lack of resolution . . . ," "break in the initial accord . . . ," "no effort . . ."), yet somehow jumps to the conclusion that the system was successful "despite this evidence." Notwithstanding the incongruity, both of the above statements were used to showcase these projects as exemplars of participatory sanitation. In contrast, the statements below, which also refer to the same two projects, were uttered by the chief of the CAERN maintenance division, who has been responsible for maintaining these projects since they were constructed. The following statements summarize a one-on-one interview I had with him in 1995.

> The Rocas condominial sewer system suffers from inadequate pipe slopes, elevations, and angles that were designed by engineers and installed by construction crews. These problems are particularly bad for homes that were built below the elevation of the street. These design and construction problems are exacerbated by the high water table and flat topography of the area, and by system misuse by the beneficiaries. Rocas has far more performance problems than any other participatory sanitation system. (Source: Informant 84, CAERN maintenance division chief and engineer, interview by the author on June 1, 1995, in Natal, Brazil)

Observe that this statement reveals a broader conception of performance and offers more sophisticated evidence that indicates poor performance or even failure, not success. I conducted a follow-up interview with this same maintenance chief in 2006, during which he made the following statement about the same two projects ten years later:

> The condominial sewer systems in Rocas and Santos Reis are still the worst performing systems in the city of Natal. (Source: Informant 84, CAERN maintenance division chief and engineer, interview by the author on January 16, 2006, in Natal, Brazil)

This analysis of a series of statements about the same projects by different types of practitioners reveals two very different perspectives about the significance of the performance problems. The engineering and finance officials who represented these projects at the national conference appeared to engage in a rhetorical use of the participatory sanitation paradigm; that is, they spoke in ways that both established and promoted the paradigm and that were supportive of the concept and the practice despite the rather obvious contradictions within their statements. As such, they played down the known performance problems and presented a narrow performance indicator that would sustain the myth of participatory sanitation. In contrast, maintenance personnel were not expected to use their specific knowledge of system performance for persuasive purposes, and as a result they were at liberty to speak materially rather than discursively about the same projects, even if only in private.

The different speech conditions and perspectives of the various actors were preserved over time by upholding a solid boundary between those who handled the systems (e.g., operations technicians and maintenance staff) and those who represented the systems (e.g., engineering and finance officials). Maintenance personnel rarely attended or spoke at Brazil's annual SANEPAR conferences, and a disciplinary separation between maintenance and engineering divisions was maintained within the organizational structures of most of Brazil's water and sanitation agencies, including CAERN. This disciplinary separation existed in spite of the fact that the CAERN maintenance chief himself was an engineer. By adopting observation methods that allowed boundary crossing and that employed symmetry in the reporting of statements (i.e., by tracing the statements of actors from a variety of disciplines and going beyond the "official" storyline), the foregoing analysis has highlighted significant contradictions in the representation of participatory sanitation and the outcome of actual projects. The discursive use of participatory sanitation by practitioners who represent the systems had the effect of validating the participatory sanitation paradigm rather than presenting any real critique or understanding of practice.

Why would practitioners engage in such rhetoric? There are several possible reasons based on different conditions of meaning. If meaning is framed by the social conditions of knowledge, then one hypothesis is that efforts to promote participatory sanitation were necessary to combat lingering resistance by other practitioners who held higher status and power because they represented conventional sanitation techniques that were socially exclusive. This resistance originally emerged in response to early condominial sewer projects, as one practitioner explains below:

> The engineers . . . didn't understand [the] proposal and some were against it but were obliged to do the work. They didn't believe in the proposal [for condominial sewers]. . . In some cases no one took responsibility [for maintenance of the public sewer]. The City didn't have the resources and the State agency did not accept the systems because *80 percent of the engineers were against the technology.* (Source: Informant 31, consulting engineer and former director of a state agency, interview by the author on March 3, 1995 in Recife, Brazil, emphasis added)

In fact, resistance to participatory sanitation was significant at first. Promotion of the approach was apparently necessary to achieve and maintain broad acceptance by sanitation practitioners and to create the space to experiment within a relatively conservative infrastructure sector. But why, after over ten years, would promotion of the participatory sanitation approach still be necessary? This state of affairs could be evidence of a continued need to defend and promote participatory development against mainstream forces.

If, on the other hand, meaning resides in the text itself rather than in experience, then practitioners who engage in rhetoric may be characterized as noncritical proponents of participatory sanitation who draw instinctively from the grand narrative of participatory development. Supporting their habitual use of participatory sanitation rhetoric is the fact that most listeners do not recognize it as myth and cannot argue against it because they lack access to practice-based, on-the-ground knowledge. Without the critical analysis of project conditions presented in the preceding chapters, one could not distinguish between these different uses of discourse, each using the same paradigm.

These findings clearly indicate that by the mid-1990s, after the initial period of innovation, a paradigm of participatory sanitation had solidified and was being used not as a theory of action or practice but as a myth to promote and extend the technology. The initial projects in Rocas and Santos Reis appear to have served as a sort of origin myth that was maintained even in the face of conflicting evidence. Actual evidence that showed mixed performance and that demonstrated the importance of the setting in which project implementation occurred was ignored in favor of a representational account that was used as if it were universally applicable in all settings. Project success stories that supported the paradigm's use as a myth were hand-picked, while project failures were unreported or misrepresented. Successes in narrow settings (e.g., small towns) were promoted for use in very different settings (e.g., capital cities) on the assumption that community participation and appropriate design were the key causal factors, as promoted by the paradigm. Successes that actually resulted from unique alignments of interest, community influence, and/or participation were instead promoted as examples of community participation and appropriate design in keeping with the paradigm. Furthermore, the knowledge and judgments of operation and maintenance (O&M) staff and of beneficiaries who lived with the projects were excluded. The dominant participatory sanitation paradigm of 1995 was therefore not an accurate portrayal of project performance during the innovation period of the previous fifteen years, it was not a useful theory of the conditions necessary for success, and it was not inclusive of the multiple narratives that existed about condominial sewers in Brazil in the 1980s and 1990s. The participatory sanitation paradigm was assumed to be objective (not subjective) and universal (not situated), and was assumed to describe the important elements of implementation everywhere, from favelas to rich neighborhoods. The participatory sanitation paradigm served as a useful myth.

A case in point is the notion that project performance was objective, when in practice performance was a subjective phenomenon. There was no standard performance measure in the mid-1990s, and performance was difficult to judge even by local condominial sewer experts. The judgments of local condominial sewer practitioners about project performance were mixed and sometimes conflicting. When asked in the context of an informal interview about all of the projects in their city, most staff (with the exception of some maintenance staff) had no difficulty and needed little prompting in identifying successful and unsuccessful projects or, when presented with a list of projects, had no difficulty placing projects from the list into good and bad categories. However, when subsequently asked to rate three or four specific projects (which I had selected) on a 5-point scale in the context of a semi-structured interview, most engineering staff responded that they did not have enough knowledge of actual project performance to provide an answer. The maintenance staff, in general, had a much more detailed and nuanced perspective on performance than the engineering, management, or social science staffs. Some maintenance staff, however, found it difficult to group projects by performance level in the context of an informal interview.[26] That project outcomes are clearly discernible, undisputed, and collectively agreed upon is one of the myths of development. In fact, different groups had different perceptions of performance, and performance outcomes were wide ranging. The only way to manage these contradictions was to limit the outcome measure down to the narrowest possible indicator (i.e., the number of connections, alternatively stated as percent coverage). An overly narrow performance measure was thus favored in lieu of a more comprehensive measure of performance. A narrow performance measure lent a sense of objectivity to the paradigm because a) the paradigm's effectiveness as a myth depended on a lack of critical analysis and a lack of thorough performance evaluation, and b) the paradigm's use was based on belief rather than on situated knowledge of real events.

By the early to mid-2000s, Melo and the World Bank had begun publishing documents that formally described the participatory sanitation narrative to the world using Brazil's condominial sewerage experience.[27] Also at this time, the World Bank published a report of its efforts to transfer the condominial approach to Bolivia, and two additional doctoral dissertations were produced (from the University of Leeds and Stanford University).[28] By this time, the participatory sanitation paradigm had evolved further, incorporating the notion of *universal service* (also called *democratization of sanitation*) as the intended performance measure. The paradigm now declared a specific (and adequately narrow) performance measure within its own statement; as in, *appropriate design and community participation lead to universal service.*

Table 7-1 presents excerpts of conference presentations by seven leading condominial sewer spokespersons (presented at a national condominial sewer conference held in Brazil[29]), which included Brazilian sanitation officials and practitioners. Within these statements, the two original pilot projects in Rocas and Santos Reis are again called out as successes on the basis of their high connection rates, suggesting that universal access had been achieved from the beginning. This is in spite of the actual poor performance quality of these two projects (as documented by maintenance staff) and despite Natal's overall low sewer connection rate. By the early 2000s, access to sewers in Natal (26 percent)[30] was only a little over half of Brazil's national average (41 percent), an outcome that was representative of the overall poor conditions in the Northeast[31] and the result of destabilization of the sanitation sector that had begun in the mid-1990s (as explained in chapter 4). By comparison, the percentage of people with access to sewer systems in Recife (43 percent)[32] had increased to just above Brazil's national average (41 percent),[33] resulting from the post-1995 consolidation of its sanitation sector (as explained in chapter 5).

The excerpts in Table 7-1 reflect the participatory sanitation paradigm of the mid-2000s. A content analysis of these excerpts yields the three key features of the paradigm at that time: 1) residents who are mobilized and ready to participate in implementation; 2) provision of universal service to communities of all income levels; and 3) design that is simple, low-cost, and appropriate (although this third element is much less prominent now than it was in earlier versions of the paradigm when appropriate technology was a more central feature). Once more, one finds a robust consensus among the messages of many different practitioners and officials, not the debate and conflict that originally surrounded condominial sewerage in the 1980s.

Although there were many other contributors, Melo and the World Bank were among the principal crafters and most influential spokespersons for the emerging global paradigm of participatory sanitation. Initially, Melo operated primarily within Brazil as a practitioner and advisor on condominial sewerage (a name that he gave the technology and the name of his engineering company); he traveled extensively throughout the country developing a reputation as a technical expert and leading promoter of the technology. Of course there were other leading spokespersons in Brazil, but Melo centered his career on the technology. There were also multiple international development agencies involved in the early experiments in condominial sewerage (including the World Bank, the UK Department for International Development, the United Nations, and the Inter-American Development Bank). But it was the World Bank that had the leading

Table 7-1. Excerpts from conference presentations by practitioners in Brazil reflecting the participatory sanitation paradigm of the mid-2000s.

Source	Excerpts[a]
Neto (2004a, 2, 3)	What differentiates and characterizes the condominial sewer model? A pattern of service directed to the majority of the population that seeks widespread sewer service. Freedom of design, a more rational layout, appropriate technology, and a better benefit-cost outcome. Community participation, a legitimate right. . . . The *condomínio* (community pact) as the unit of collection, which facilitates collective solutions, decisions, and participatory management. What's more, the model promotes the democratic principles of gradualism, progressivism, sanitary security, environmental sustainability, social justice, economic scale, articulated action, forces, implementation, and community participation.
Lobo (2004, 10) Bolivia	The proposition is for community participation in construction and maintenance of condominial sewer connections, presenting a new model of management that we call participatory management between the operator and the *condomínios*.
Miranda (2004, 33)	Requirements for universalization (of sanitation service): national sanitation policy, planning, investment programs, adequate regulation of services with social control, participation of the population.
Nazareth (2004, 5, 9, 40–42)	Objective of the model: the universalization of service. Logic of the model: "*those who perceive of a problem are natural agents of the solution . . . this solution must result from a pact among those interested.*" Key idea of the model: democratization of services through information, decision-making, and access. A condominial meeting is a moment of participation, negotiation, decision-making, and promotion of the community organization. This moment is an accord between the users and the implementer of the service seeking a solution to the local sanitation problem. Critical aspects in employment of the condominial model: political decision, knowledge of the model, institutional incorporation, adequate rules, qualification of the implementer, adequate design/construction/use/operation, and sustainability. Institutional requirements for its implementation: political adoption of the condominial system and desired level of community participation.
Rissoli (2004, 4, 16, 17, 19)	The objective of the Federal District's Condominial Sewer Program is universalization of sewer service and social development. The basic component of the model is community mobilization, community participation is the objective and condominial meetings are the central element. The results of a condominial meeting are: to organize an informal *condomínio*, to democratize information, to decide about the best form of sewer service for the *condomínio*, to elect a union representative, and to discuss the notion of sanitary education. Participation leads to 100 percent connection to the system. The adoption of the Condominial Model as the single alternative for rich and poor neighborhoods was the fundamental element of success in the experience of the Federal District.

Source	Excerpts[a]
Carvalho (2004:33, 35)	[There is a] lack of involvement and participation of the population due to a lack of culture and organized community practice and lack of public services. [These can be solved by doing the following:]: a) recruitment of community representatives to help the social work staff mobilize residents, b) identification of community leaders, c) prioritizing the implementation of projects in well-organized communities, d) ______, e) creating a position for assessing project quality, and f) installation of telephones exclusively for complaints, with operators specialized in the resolution of problems. [There are several difficulties in the] formation of *condomínios*: a) necessity for a minimum quorum of 50% plus 1 residents present at the meeting to establish a condomínio, b) election of a union leader and sub-union leader to represent the condomínio, and c) minimum __% percent of residents per block must agree to sign the contract in order to realize the project. [These can be solved by doing the following:] a) intensification of social work, including house to house visits, b) changing the hours of the project meetings so that they coincide with the reality of the community, c) a union school as desired by the community.
Mariz (2004: 17, 23-24, 26-27)	Caixa Economica Federal was involved in a cooperative development program modeled on decentralized management of the implementation of basic sanitation in Brazil—the PROSAB Program. Condominial Model of Rio Grande do Norte: CAERN—condominial work group—research on alternatives for sanitary sewerage in low-income areas . . . conventional project. The conventional solution predicted to serve 30% of the population. The pilot experience in Rocas and Santos Reis (block 90)—a condominial sewer—was approved by practitioners, the population, the World Bank, and the Bank of Brazil. Results: implementation of 2884 condominial sewer connections and 420 individual sewer connections—97% coverage– drying out the area from standing sewage. Condominial Model in Practice: incorporated into CAIXA's appropriate technology programs that produce economical and efficient solutions......actually considered as a model for solutions in diverse urban areas regardless of the income of the population. Condominial Model: stimulates action and integrated management of urban services that induce empowerment through community participation. This model can contribute as an instrument for implementing public policy that results in the universalization of environmental sanitation services, and which acts as an agent of effective change in the life of the population.

a. Translations by the author (with some unknown phrases left blank).

role in funding many of the initial condominial sewer projects that were implemented during the International Water and Sanitation Decade (1980–1990), that published much of the literature on the topic, that had the ability to reach a global audience, and that consequently embraced the leading role in developing and distributing a global participatory sanitation paradigm, almost without critique. By the early to mid-2000s, condominial sewerage and the participatory sanitation paradigm were no longer controversial; the debates had subsided and the technology and its paradigm had become objectified.

Innovation and the Socio-Material Dialectic

Perspective is the privilege of those standing at a distance in time and space from actual events—it is a new frame of reference, a new context. Those who are there inside the action do not know which of their deeds, acts, or events will later become historically significant. In Bruno Latour's words, scientists and engineers often proceed "based on decisions about an uncertain future, rather than on logical deductions from past events."[34] Their criteria for right action are unknown, arbitrary, or underdetermined. The collective creation of a discourse about participatory sanitation by activist engineers took place within these conditions. The activist engineers did not know how condominial sewers would be received or whether participation would become accepted; some aspects of the discourse certainly did not follow logically from the performance outcomes of the early projects. They did recognize they were innovating,[35] that they were engaged in politics (in addition to engineering), and that their statements had to have the power to *enroll* new supporters[36] (i.e., to attract allies) in order to win the battle over the frame of reference for speaking about sewers. These conditions required the instrumental use of myth.

In addition to having the benefit of recent historical perspective, our examination will include an understanding of how facts (and discourses) were constructed *as* they were constructed, and how they were made to give the effect of objectivity—in this case, how activist engineers started with an array of unsubstantiated statements and ideas and ended up with a new consolidated object that would eventually spread to other developing countries and make possible the widespread adoption of condominial sewerage. These unsubstantiated statements—i.e., the circa-1995 paradigm, after what we can now see as the end of the 1980–1995 innovation period—were designed to overcome the tide of social exclusion and bias within the conventional sanitation sector. The activist engineers and their allies were creating a social movement. Today when someone speaks of condominial sewers they are referring to a way of thinking that can now be explained, defined, and specified in a more or less consistent manner, no matter what the physical project ends up looking like or who is speaking. This consistency in a way of thinking was not always there; rather, it is the effect to be explained.

Early in what can now be understood as the recent history of participatory sanitation, there was no agreement about what "participatory sanitation" was. On the contrary, there was heated debate about what the new technology was or should be, about its efficiency and effectiveness, and about who it should serve and how it should be implemented. Resistance to condominial sewer technology was particularly strong from engineers who supported conventional sewer technology. One might expect to find that the early condominial sewer experiments were so successful that engineers from one city to another accepted and adopted the new technology on the basis of actual performance outcomes, making the emergence and diffusion of the participation sanitation paradigm a quite rational and linear process. But that is simply not the case. The new technology was *not* consistently successful and certain very rare conditions were necessary for its success. In some settings, such as Recife, failure was much more common than success. So the question remains, how is it that the notion of participatory sanitation became widely accepted, incorporated into Brazil's sewer design standards, counted as an object in the Brazilian census, and embraced by international development agencies for replication around the world? To explain this effect, we must turn to the arguments of Bruno Latour and his actor-network theory.

In 1979, Bruno Latour published a groundbreaking book called *Laboratory Life: The Construction of Scientific Facts*. In that book he spelled out the beginnings of a new argument about how scientific facts get created by scientists in laboratories. Over a series of subsequent books,[37] Latour and other scholars from diverse disciplines, including the history and philosophy of science and science and technology studies, fully developed an actor-oriented approach to the analysis of scientific controversies and technological innovations. By way of introduction, I will attempt a brief summary of one aspect of the approach—that being the theory of fact construction—applied to sewer technology, simply to elucidate the complex questions being asked and to provide a critical stance from which to view the subsequent analysis.

In the so-called first world, conventional sewer technology has become mundane and so unproblematic that it is rarely even discussed (except among experts). It is easy to forget that there once was a time (in the 1800s and early 1900s) when what would become conventional sewers were at the center of public health and urban development debates.[38] There was a time when sewer technology was an untried and experimental technology, and when the opinions of influential non-technical people mattered just as much, if not more so, than the statements of leading engineers and physicians. Because there was yet no basis for objectivity, *who* was speaking mattered, as the personal credibility of the person speaking could lend credibility and thus objectivity about the new notion of sewers, even before sewers had reached the status of an object.[39] Sewers, then, were once a subject of political discourse, not the solidified object of today's engineering circles. Today, in the usual situation where conventional sewer technology does not pose a problem, it does not generally matter who I am when I describe a sewer. My status now has no bearing on the objective (or unsituated) description of a sewer because today sewers have been made to exist as objects and there is now widespread agreement on what an accurate representational account looks like. The hydraulic and structural knowledge behind their design now exists as a set of uncontroversial, depoliticized facts, and statements made about sewer objects that mimic the representational norm will be largely uncontested and viewed as objective (except in rare instances where debates still exist). Every infrastructure textbook contains very similar descriptions, or unsituated representations, of sewer technology stripped of its historical time and place, and just about everyone would fall back on such descriptions when trying to describe a sewer today (although the language might need to be adjusted to different audiences). These representations typically contain no contextual information, and it is this act of de-contextualizing and de-situating that is essential to the construction and ultimate solidification of facts and objects themselves. As the diversity of representations converge and as debates subside, the original subject being described eventually achieves the status of a solidified fact or object whose existence is unquestioned. How it achieved that status is no longer important, that is, unless a problem arises that restarts the debate.[40]

But when debates are still active, it is essential to know to whom one is speaking. For example, the quote that opened this chapter cannot be properly interpreted without understanding when it was said and who said it. If the quote was uttered at a time when participatory sanitation/condominial sewerage was not yet solidified into a single uncontroversial representational account (ca. 1980s), then the statement has no "objective" standing because it only represents the conjecture, belief, or rhetoric of the speaker, who only stands for him- or herself and not for the "objective facts" (since the facts have yet to be determined or objectified as facts). At this early stage of their existence, the "sociomaterial character" of condominial sewers and the "complex interdependencies between people and things" (to use Stephen Healy's terms) are perceptible.[41] Most likely the speaker is one of the activist engineers involved in the condominial sewer movement.

But if the opening quote was uttered in the 2000s, at a time when participatory sanitation/condominial sewerage was no longer controversial, then we would more likely interpret the same very statement as "pure" factual information, and we would perceive the very same statement to be objective no matter who uttered it, ignoring that we are drawing from an imagined realm of technological and scientific "truth" that has been made to be separate from context and speaker. If we point out that it was an engineer who said it, it would be to lend even more "facticity" to the statement based on the assumption that engineers represent not themselves but "objective" facts, systems, and machines, and that engineers typically delete for us any "nonessential subjectivity"—it would not be to criticize the statement. Consequently, the existence of an object is relative[42] (i.e., it may range from a mutable and contested idea in the 1980s to a completely solidified object in the 2000s), and its facticity is a function of time, place, and who is speaking; however the interdependency between the social and material aspects of objects is only recognized (if at all) when the proposed object is unsolidified, surrounded in controversy, or interpreted as fiction, such as during the initial period of innovation of a new technology.

These actor-oriented (or object-oriented) conceptual distinctions allow us to ask questions about the interdependency between statements and objects, their shades of existence at various points in time and space, the nature of the gap between the social (i.e., participatory sanitation discourse) and the material (i.e., condominial sewer projects), and the discursive aspects of material objects. These concepts allow us to trace not only the difference between what people say about development and the actual outcomes of development (i.e., the smaller questions about development practice), they allow us to observe the battle for control over the frame of reference in which objects and outcomes are described (i.e., the larger questions about knowledge and power), such as the perceived legitimacy of the engineer's point of view versus that of maintenance workers or lay people. Most importantly, it allows us to accept the necessity of the gap between the participatory sanitation paradigm and the variety of situated objects called condominial sewer projects, as well as the gap in discourse between practitioners who serve as spokespeople for innovation in action and practitioners who do not. I might go so far as to say that if outcomes on the ground were the only driving force for adopting new technology, then participatory sanitation would probably never have achieved its current status because there would have been no way to cope with the necessary failures of the innovation period, and there would have been no way to manage the transition from myth to object (i.e., the socio-material dialectic).

Participation as Ethno-development

Why was it necessary for engineers—known for their so-called objectivity—to speak of the social aspects of condominial sewers rather than the material aspects; that is, why did they use the participatory sanitation paradigm as a myth? Perlman (1976) showed the poverty paradigm as a myth, inaccurate in its description of poor people and resulting in misrepresentation and othering. Feachem (1980) revealed the participatory sanitation paradigm as a myth that did not accurately portray the actual conditions of development's successes and failures in the water and sanitation sector; and argued that its use as a myth distracted from practice-based understanding. My ethnographies of condominial sewer projects in Natal and Recife (presented in chapter 6) also showed that the participatory sanitation paradigm did not explain outcomes of specific projects as accurately as project coalition theory; that community participation provided only partial information about the conditions that lead to success and failure; and that the community participation narrative marginalized competing narratives. Feachem's nearly thirty-year-old warning has gone unheeded and the participatory sanitation paradigm has never been stronger. So, then, why are myths constructed, whom do they serve, and what is their functional role in development?

Myth can be viewed as a form of speech that is used to enroll spokespeople and bind them together as a network,[43] and the myth does not have to be empirically accurate to be effective. Participatory sanitation myth serves to hold together condominial sewerage as a technology within the water and sanitation sector. It also serves to attract new spokespeople who are compelled by its ethical and humanitarian impulse and/or by its moment of deconstruction of the existing power relations in society. But maintaining the myth has meant eluding critique and avoiding a larger deconstruction of the power relations of participation, an aspect of Grillo and Stirrat's (1997) epistemological trap. The participatory sanitation paradigm is used not only to enroll new spokespeople; it provides the assumed framework in which projects are evaluated, thereby setting up a context that excludes some narratives and some actions from consideration and that pre-frames the discussion so as to limit critical analysis of the paradigm. This is why there was no space for critical evaluation and critique during fact construction, why the maintenance of an origin myth was important, why there was almost unanimous agreement (rather than debate) among spokespeople, and why there was constant repetition of the same key features of the paradigm (as expressed in the statements in Table 7-1) rather than multiple perspectives and narratives. Questions about performance quality at the individual project level and the appropriation of labor via participation were out of bounds; and the perspectives of project beneficiaries and O&M technicians were obscured (unless they supported the paradigm). The paradigm over-relied on formal government-designed forms of participation, while uncontrolled forms of collective action performed for the purpose of aligning interests and increasing community influence were not counted as participation as defined by the paradigm. Without the balance of real critique and evaluation, the spokespeople for participatory sanitation ended up promoting a myth that served to hide its own existence as a myth, because once viewed as a myth its positive power to enroll is removed. The conditions of fact construction depend on maintaining a divide between myth and critique.

There were clear advantages to constructing a participatory sanitation paradigm and using it as a myth for promoting condominial sewerage: these actions mobilized countless spokespeople to focus on the needs of the poor, thereby catalyzing real innovation. This necessary period of descriptive story building in a context of controversy required the avoidance of accurate critiques and descriptions of practice, which went largely unnoticed and unchecked within and among spokespeople. There was no space within paradigm construction for critical material discussions such as the one I have carried out in this book. Consequently, the instrumental use of story as a constructive and necessary aspect of innovation was discursively suppressed (also a condition of fact construction). And even though the participatory sanitation narrative was constructive and necessary for innovation, as I am arguing, it is not sufficient in the long term to stabilize the project coalition networks that produce successful outcomes. If the innovation is to endure, there should be a transition from story to theory whereby the participatory sanitation paradigm becomes part of "regular' development theory and subject to critique that problematizes development itself.[44] If the innovation of participatory sanitation occurred primarily during the years 1980 to 1995, then we are now in the post-innovation period where participatory sanitation vies to become sanitation in an un-"othered" form. The post-innovation period presents an opportunity to shift from thinking separately about the needs of previously unserved populations to including them automatically in everyday development practice—in short, allowing the previously excluded to join the collective. If successful—and success is not guaranteed—then this new form of conventional sanitation (itself once an innovation instead of a convention) would be more inclusive than previous forms; it would be larger in scope and contain more diversity. If this transition is successful, then some aspect of the promise of participatory development (from chapter 1) would have been achieved.

The transition we are now in, from innovation to inclusion, will require more than the construction of paradigms-as-myth to be successful. Interactions between the social and the material will now have to be viewed as *matters of fact* (to use Latour's term) if they are to endure over the long term, thus requiring the construction of paradigms-as-theory. In other words, participatory sanitation will have to be tested by scientific means. It will have to undergo trials, real critique, and critical evaluation from multiple perspectives, just as development itself has. The gloves must come off. Of course, Brazil's conventional sanitation sector was very critical of condominial technology from the beginning, yet they had no viable approach for extending service to non-elite population segments, and their critique came off as a thinly veiled attempt to maintain a status quo in which they had control over the frame of reference and dominance of the sector. This is not the kind of critical evaluation I am suggesting. I am arguing for a critical evaluation that includes multi-stakeholder evaluations of project performance (i.e., where the voices and perspectives of residents, operators, maintenance technicians, and others usually excluded from infrastructure evaluation are meaningfully included side-by-side with the voices and perspectives of traditional actors—engineers, sanitation officials, and other conventional spokespeople) and that is inclusive of diverse needs and circumstances.[45] This kind of critique would be intended to make condominial sewer networks even more durable and more inclusive—and we now understand that the term "networks" refers simultaneously to physical pipe networks and project coalition networks. This book has offered a partial demonstration of a critique of participatory sanitation based on critical ethnographies of practice.

Despite the necessary myth of the participatory sanitation paradigm, the construction of the paradigm had a functional role, which was to inspire, attract, and facilitate the formation of groups specifically interested in including poor people in development. Just as the artificiality of laboratories that are constructed to showcase specific experimental results in no way taints the perceived objectiveness of the scientific facts that emerge from them, the myth of participatory sanitation motivated a critical mass of spokespeople around a shared subject and eventually effected real objective changes in Brazil's water and sanitation sector. These changes included new sewer system design standards, expansions in service, and new expectations for the role of residents in infrastructure development. The activist engineers did indeed win the battle for a new sanitation framework that included the poor, thereby fulfilling part of the promise of participatory development. But if the networks they helped establish are to endure and expand further, their objects must hold up to trials of critical evaluation done with the awareness that myth and subjectivity are implicated in the construction of development projects.

Having already offered (in chapter 6) a set of ethnographic observation methods that focused attention on the unique circumstances, situated actions, and viewpoints of a range of local actors in their settings (i.e., project ethnographies), and a set of maps of the actor-networks associated with particular projects under specific conditions (i.e., project coalitions), this last analysis brings us to what I hope is the ultimate accomplishment of the book: a new account of development that acknowledges social networks and projects emerging simultaneously.

The early experiments in sanitary sewerage were quite controversial and were the subject of great political and social debate as well as techno-scientific controversy by a wide array of individuals. Everything about sanitation was in formation. Through many conflicts and trials, the networks that produced sanitary sewerage became less controversial, more durable, and were eventually made to work more efficiently by adopting more actors into the network, such as new laws, routines, and standards, which did some of the work of holding project coalitions together. In time, some of the "net"-work done by these diverse actors became invisible as the material aspects were made to be seen as separate from the social aspects, and the physical output—the sewer system—became solidified as a techno-scientific object now known as conventional sanitation. Today, all references to conventional sanitation refer primarily to objects in their final physical form, not to the years of involvement by multitudes of hybrid actors building the networks from which these objects were born. The networks have become invisible and only the sewer systems are visible.

Conventional development projects are spoken of as solidified objects (hence their conventionality), and the project coalitions that sustain them have been made invisible in discourse. As a result, conventional development projects (such as conventional sanitation systems) are not considered "participatory"—the social aspect has been removed. But in practice, these projects emerge from the participation of many human and non-human actors. At the same time, there are "other" versions of sanitation that are called participatory, where the social aspect is still recognized. In these versions, it is possible to observe the project coalitions as they are being constructed. The social aspects of the technology are still recognized, the physical aspects are still being formed, and people are doing much of the work themselves. Regardless of which version of sanitation is being discussed (conventional or participatory), it is the nature and quality of the project coalition/actor-network that produces the outcome. Each project is performed or acted out by a project coalition that is observable only in practice, emergent of specific times and places, and the work of many actors; in other words, each project is an ethno-development.

In many ways, the course of action hypothesized above is similar to the process that people in the Global South are going through today—they are beginning to create their sanitation networks, many with the benefit of condominial sewer technology. In the minority world of the Global North, these sanitation networks have been solidified for years and the work to maintain them is (usually) no longer done only by direct participation of people; it is done by many types of non-human actors (e.g., laws, standards, routines, organizations, technologies, machines, etc.). The maps of these project coalitions would be far more complex than the simple maps I developed for a handful of condominial sewer projects. Despite this, we do not call conventional projects "participatory" because the work done by human and non-human actors to maintain the project coalitions is discursively denied, as Latour predicted, and the social component has been obscured. Hence, conventional sanitation is largely perceived as an engineering object with a limited social component. It is easier to recognize participatory sanitation as ethno-development, with the social still visibly tied-up with the scientific and the technical; in fact, both conventional and participatory sanitation are ethno-developments held together by project coalitions.

By acknowledging networks (i.e., project coalitions) we follow the principle of symmetry to reconstruct both participatory development and conventional development as ethno-development (in its most positive connotation); that is, as an emergent, performative process in which actors respond to and manipulate pressures and opportunities in accordance with their own drives and knowledges, where some innovations are eventually solidified into objects, and where over time certain networks are made to be more stable than others. We should not expect project development outcomes to be explained by the paradigms from which their objects emerge, since we now recognize the existence of a socio-material dialectic and the positive function of myth in making the collective more inclusive. And we now recognize the positive role of critical evaluation in making development objects and development networks more durable.

Closing Remarks for Chapter 7

This chapter analyzed how the participatory sanitation paradigm and (subsequently) condominial sewer projects evolved and transformed over time. The promoters of condominial sewer technology distilled their diverse ideas and experiences into a general model or paradigm of participatory sanitation. This paradigm was identified through a content analysis of texts (written and oral) used by the engineers and sanitation officials who carried, altered, and narrated the paradigm. In their efforts to promote the adoption of condominial sewers throughout Brazil, the originator of the approach (José Carlos Melo) and his allies asserted that participation in an "association of households" (known in Brazil as a *condomínio*) was important to the success of condominial sewer projects; that is, that better participation led to better project outcomes. The expressed rationale for participatory sanitation was fundamentally the same as the more general paradigm of participatory development; however, the participatory sanitation paradigm inspired but did not accurately predict or describe real project experiences that occurred during the innovation period (1980–1995). The promoters had an overwhelmingly positive orientation and non-critical attitude toward participatory sanitation, which was necessary to their effectiveness as spokespeople who persuaded other engineers and sanitation officials to adopt the technology. The paradigm of participatory sanitation was used discursively, rather than empirically, to manage contradictions between idealized outcomes and actual project outcomes, and to create and maintain consensus about the validity of the paradigm itself. Managing contradictions and maintaining consensus were important for enrollment purposes; that is, for the purpose of attracting others who would be inspired to join the network of spokespeople for the innovative technology.

Today, Brazil is using the participatory sanitation paradigm to extend condominial sewer services to more of its population. In terms of the number of people served—the only performance measure currently in widespread use—project experiences after the innovation period have improved tremendously compared to the earlier project outcomes. Nevertheless, promoters continue to highlight some of the initial condominial sewer projects from the innovation period as exemplars in spite of their consistently low-grade performance over three decades. And a standard method for evaluating project performance in a more comprehensive manner has still not caught on. Motivated by an ethical impulse that views participation as always positive and beneficial, the participatory sanitation paradigm continues to be used to validate an orthodox participatory development paradigm and to enroll new adopters, thus impeding any real critique of the phenomenon in practice. This raises questions for how Brazil's unique experiment with participatory sanitation should be studied. Studies that take as their point of departure the assumption that this experiment was monolithically positive are part of the problem to be solved. Critical evaluative research is needed to displace the privileged stance implied by such assumptions.

Overall Conclusions

Condominial sewers hold a central and important place in international development. They meet the needs and tenets of the dominant discourse of development and contribute to the ideology of participatory development. Indeed, they have contributed to the mainstreaming of participation and appropriate technology in the sanitation sector, and they can be responsive to the objective conditions of many people in the developing world and thereby legitimate the notion that participatory development is necessary and beneficial. However, in the early development stages of condominial sewers the experiences on the ground were mixed—characterized by failure and dissatisfaction in some places and by success in others. Urban residents experienced poor to moderate performance and low to moderate satisfaction with both the systems and the participation process.

The book developed a theory of project coalitions by applying the methods of ethnography to condominial sewer projects. The theory was useful in characterizing how successful and failed projects emerged during Brazil's initial innovation period. The project coalition account explained actual outcomes better than the dominant paradigm (which stated that participation and appropriate design lead to good performance). Nevertheless, Brazil has widely adopted a participatory sanitation paradigm for the development of urban sewer projects and is now extending the paradigm to water systems with increasing success. Curiously, this proliferation of participatory projects has not relied on critical evaluations of actual project performance, but on increasingly polished discursive use of the participatory sanitation paradigm as an expression of a more broadly based participatory development model. Promoters of condominial sewers, mostly engineers, marginalized real outcomes and used the paradigm of participatory sanitation to "explain" how success was achieved. The process, known as the theory of fact construction, required the repression of deeper critiques of projects installed under the new paradigm, as well as marginalization of competing narratives held by residents and maintenance staffs. The paradigm was attractive to those seeking funding from the World Bank and other international lenders who promoted participatory development worldwide through their projects. And it was attractive to people who desperately wanted and sought solutions to their objective sanitation conditions, conditions which had been exacerbated by the negative effects of modern development itself. The process of the origination and spread of condominial sewers in Brazil played a role in the global mainstreaming of participatory development by the World Bank

For all of these reasons, we can understand why a gap was maintained between the participatory sanitation paradigm (i.e., the social) and on-the-ground development outcomes (i.e., the material) during the period of innovation. To be effective, it appears that maintaining this gap required a necessarily vague conception of development based on an overly narrow indicator of performance (as opposed to situated in-depth analyses of performance), and a necessarily noncritical attitude about participation. All of the observations in the book are therefore unified by the idea that development innovation does not result from objective evaluation of (or even learning from) real outcomes; but rather is a consequence of collective myth-making about how development is achieved, followed by subsequent technological improvements that may or may not impact the paradigm. In other words, development has a significant narrative aspect whose purpose is to create space for technological experimentation. Successful narration of the participatory sanitation paradigm opened the way for a period of trial and error that eventually led to more successful projects and, eventually, a complete transformation of Brazil's water and sanitation sector. While controversial at first, this way of thinking is now part of mainstream development theory and practice, in which condominial sewers are considered a local example of a larger model of participatory development, and where project outcomes are often understood in terms of this model. Further consolidation of condominial sewer technology will require real critique by evaluators who are aware of the role of the socio-material dialectic in innovations and who acknowledge that all projects—participatory or conventional—are the work of multiple actors maintaining networks.

Today, participatory sanitation is the norm in many of Brazil's municipalities, with some cities performing exceptionally well[46] and successfully serving a majority of their residents with condominial sewer systems. Expansion of condominial sewers in Brazil is now being tracked officially by the national census, and the World Bank and others are taking the innovation to other developing countries who are dealing with the problems of social exclusion in their water and sanitation sectors. These are extraordinarily positive developments compared to practices of the recent past whereby the state, with impunity, either ignored the needs of the poor or carried out organized aggression against their autonomy. This real success would not have been possible without the collective construction of a participatory sanitation paradigm and its successful use as a myth to attract a vast network of actors engaged in transforming sanitation.

Notes

1. This statement was made by a condominial sewer practitioner who was interviewed by the author in Natal in 1995.

2. The notion of a *condomínio*, also broadly known as a user group, is distinct from the notion of a project coalition. A condomínio would be considered one actor among several that make up a project coalition. Condomínio*s* did not always form in practice, however.

3. Although there is a growing literature on *esgoto condominiais* (often translated into English as "condominial sewers"), I use two terms in my analysis. I use the term "condominial sewer" to signify a category of physical infrastructure systems that as a group are different from conventional sewer systems in specific ways. I use the term "participatory sanitation" to refer to the (now global) discursive practices and ideas surrounding condominial sewerage that link it directly with broader discourses on participation and development. The word "participatory" makes clear reference to community participation, one of the fundamental principles of condominial sewers; whereas the word "condominial," literally referring to a condominium building, remains culturally and historically distinct within Brazil. The Brazilian originators of condominial sewerage adopted the word "condominial" because of the perceived similitude between a system of horizontal pipes that collected sewage from homes on the same block and a system of vertical pipes that collected sewage from Brazil's high-rise condominiums and apartment buildings. If the vertical sewer system in a condominium building were laid horizontally down the middle of a city block, it would serve the same purpose and have a similar physical appearance as a condominial sewer. Despite the original reference to Brazilian condominiums, the opening quote of this chapter reveals that physical layout is not a defining feature of condominial systems even though the name has stuck. Using the word "participatory" (instead of "condominial") in my analysis removes any reference to the physical features of a horizontal condominium and provides a technical term for the intended meaning of condominial sewers, which is collective service to a group of homes whose

residents participate in service provision. For the second term, I use the word "sanitation" (instead of "sewer") to encompass 1) the sewage collection function of a condominial sewer, 2) the sewage treatment and storage functions of a septic tank typically attached to a condominial sewer, and 3) the sanitary practices of residents involved in operating and maintaining a condominial sewer. Furthermore, because many neighborhoods had no public trunk sewer to which they could connect their condominial sewer, many neighborhoods discharged into local septic tanks which were considered part of a decentralized condominial sewer system. It is unclear whether such hybrid systems should be considered small-scale sewer systems (where the "scale" is a number of blocks or a group of homes instead of an entire drainage basin) or large-scale onsite sanitation systems (where the "site" is the neighborhood instead of an individual lot); nevertheless the broader term sanitation incorporates all of these sewage management functions. To summarize, I use the term "participatory sanitation" to refer to discursive practices about condominial sewers as a social construct, and I use the term "condominial sewer" to refer to specific projects in the ground that are locally known as condominial sewer projects no matter what the physical layout is or whether people actually participated.

4. See for example, World Bank (1994 and 2004) and the United Nations (2005).

5. An earlier form of decentralization based on regional economic growth that swept across Brazil and other Latin American states in the pre-World War II period is, in hindsight, now seen as a failure (Campbell, 2003, 9).

6. World Bank, 1994, 75; and World Bank, 2004, 29, 89; also see Ostrom, 1996; Allison, 2002; Lemos and Looye, 2003; Joshi and Moore, 2004; Kulipossa, 2004; and Pearce, 2004.

7. World Bank, 1994, 76, and World Bank, 2004, 9; also see IRC, no date; Korten, 1980; Paul, 1987; Oakley et al., 1991; Briscoe and Garn, 1995; Narayan, 1995; Chambers, 1997; Goetz and Gaventa, 2001; Lemos et al., 2002; Meshack, 2004; Moran and Batley, 2004; and Lavalle et al., 2005

8. World Bank, 1994, 82; and World Bank, 2004, 25; also see Solo et al., 1993; Bell and Franceys, 1995; Watson and Jagannathan, 1995; Feachem, McGarry, and Mara, 1977; Vines, Reed, and Pickford, 1990; Sinnatamby, 1990; and UNDP, 2003.

9. The earlier appropriate technology era of the 1960s and 1970s is now often characterized as a disappointment (Goethert, 2005 and Fisher, 2004).

10. See, for example, Ferguson, 1990; Escobar, 1992 and 1995; Sachs (ed.). 1992; Hobart (ed.), 1993; Grillo and Stirrat (eds.), 1997; Rahnema and Bawtree (eds.), 1997; Esteva and Prakash (eds.), 1998; Scott, 1999; and Parfitt, 2002.

11. Hobart (ed.), 1993,5.

12. Grillo and Stirrat (eds.), 1997, 26–27 cite exemplary studies by Pigg, 1992; Harrison, 1995; and Long, 1992.

13. See, for example, Grillo and Stirrat (eds.), 1997; Preston, 1994; Marsden, 1994; Gardner, 1997; Seddon, 1993; and Hobart (ed.), 1993.

14. See Hobart (ed.), 1993, 12.

15. See Nance, 2005.

16. See, for example: Perlman, 1976 (*The Myth of Marginality*); Feachem, 1980 (Community Participation in Appropriate Water Supply and Sanitation Technologies: The Mythology for the Decade); Bauzon (ed.), 1992 *(Development and Democratization in the Third World: Myths, Hopes and Realities*); Weiss, 1998 (*The Myth of the Powerless State*); Ferguson, 1999 (*Expectations of Modernity: Myths and Meanings of Urban Life on the Zambian Copperbelt*); International Organization for Migration, 2006 (*Mi-*

grants Remittances and Development: Myths, Rhetoric and Realities); and Yi-chong and Weller, 2009 (*Inside the World Bank: Exploding the Myth of the Monolithic Bank*).

17. The questions I am asking about engineers and development projects draw from the questions that Bruno Latour asked about scientists and laboratories (see *Laboratory Life: The Construction of Scientific Facts*, 1979, 31–36).

18. See, for example, Bakalian, Wright, Otis, and Azevedo-Netto, 1993; Bakalian and Jagannathan, 1991; Azevedo-Netto, 1988; Melo, 1985; Neto and Filho, 1985; Neto, Medeiros, and Melo, 1983; and Sinnatamby, 1983.

19. See Melo 1994, published by Caixa Econômica Federal.

20. Gabrielle Watson, "Good Sewers Cheap?: Agency-Customer Interactions in Low-Cost Urban Sanitation in Brazil," *Water and Sanitation Currents, UNDP-World Bank Water and Sanitation Program* (Washington, DC: The World Bank, 1995).

21. Watson and Jagannathan, 1995.

22. See, for example, Melo, 1994; Mara, 1996; Cairncross and Feachem, 1993; and Pickford, 1995.

23. Sources, in the order presented, are condominial sewer practitioners from Natal (Informants 75, 87, 89, 96, 120, and 121) and from Recife (Informants 1, 3, 7, 9, 12, 29, and 59), interviewed by the author in 1994 and 1995. See references for bibliographic information on each informant.

24. Personal communication with Jesse Motta Carvalho Filho, Director of Operations at Empresa Baiana de Águas e Saneamento (EMBASA), Salvador, Bahia, January 30, 2006.

25. See Nance (2005) and Nance and Ortolano (2007) for a more detailed analysis of participation versus performance for the projects in Natal and Recife. Only the broad results of this analysis are summarized here.

26. See Nance (2005 and 2004, ch. 3) for a more complete discussion of this topic. Only the broad results are reported here.

27. See Melo 2005, published by the World Bank.

28. See Foster, n.d.; Sarmento, 2002; and Nance, 2004.

29. SANEPAR Congress, Curitiba, Brazil, September 1-2, 2004.

30. Access to piped water in Natal (97 percent) exceeded Brazil's national average (84 percent) during the 1999 to 2000 timeframe.

31. These calculations use data from IBGE. Sources are World Factbook, http://www.odci.gov/cia/publications/factbook/geos/br.html; IBGE, http://www.IBGE.gov.br, 2001; IBGE PNAD, 1999; IBGE *Anuário Estatístico do Brasil*, 1992; IBGE *Censo Demográfico 2000—Malha Municipal Digital do Brasil*, 1997; http://www.ibge.gov.br/cidadesat; Populstat, http://www.library.uu.nl/wesp/populstat/Americas/brazilc.htm, 2003; World Bank, 1994; Parlatore, undated; and Informant 79, CAERN planning division chief, interview by author, 24 April 1995, Natal, transcript.

32. Access to piped water in Recife (88 percent) exceeded Brazil's national average (84 percent) during the 1999 to 2000 timeframe.

33. These calculations use data from IBGE. Sources are World Factbook, http://www.odci.gov/cia/publications/factbook/geos/br.html; IBGE, http://www.ibge.gov.br, 2001; IBGE PNAD, 1999; IBGE *Anuário Estatístico do Brasil*, 1992; IBGE *Censo Demográfico 2000—Malha Municipal Digital do Brasil*, 1997; http://www.ibge.gov.br/cidadesat; Populstat, http://www.library.uu.nl/wesp/populstat/Americas/brazilc.htm, 2003; World Bank, 1994; World Bank, 2003; and Parlatore, undated.

34. See Bruno Latour, *Laboratory Life: The Construction of Scientific Facts*, page 116.

35. Two veteran practitioners from Recife whom I interviewed in 1995 declared the previous fifteen years as "a series of demonstration projects" undertaken by the City "to disseminate condominial sewer technology" and "to show COMPESA how to resolve the sanitation problem." (Informant 3, EMLURB official, interview by author, March 13, 1995, Recife, transcript; and Informant 7, URB department chief, interview by author, March 8, 1995, Recife, transcript).

36. See Latour, 1987, 108.

37. See especially: *Science in Action: How to Follow Scientists and Engineers through Society* (1987), *The Pasteurization of France* (1988), *We Have Never Been Modern* (1993), *Pandora's Hope: Essays on the Reality of Science Studies* (1999), *Politics of Nature: How to Bring the Sciences into Democracy* (2004), *and Reassembling the Social* (2005).

38. The social/political/technological/scientific history of early sewerage and sanitation is covered in books by Joel Tarr (*The Search for the Ultimate Sink: Urban Pollution in Historical Perspective*) and Bruno Latour (*The Pasteurization of France*).

39. Bruno Latour has demonstrated that there is no such thing as an objective stance from which to judge the facticity of statements (see *Science in Action*, 27).

40. These are, broadly, the arguments put forth by Bruno Latour in *Laboratory Life* (1979) and *Science in Action* (1987), applied to sewer technology.

41. Stephen Healy introduces the terms "socio-material character" and "complex interdependencies between people and things" in the article "Toward a Vocabulary for Speaking of the Engagement of Things into Discourse," *Journal of Environmental Policy and Planning* 7, no. 3 (September 2005), 239–56. In this article, Healy also provides an excellent overview of Latour's philosophy.

42. Bruno Latour introduces the concept of the "relative existence" of objects in the book *Pandora's Hope: Essays on the Reality of Science Studies*, 156.

43. This argument draws from a broader argument made by Bruno Latour about the process of enrollment and the formation of groups around constructed objects (see *Reassembling the Social*, 2005, 27–42).

44. See Grillo and Stirrat, 1997, 27.

45. See Nance, 2005 for an example of multi-stakeholder evaluation.

46. Brazil's national capital of Brasilia is a good example of recent condominial sewer success, which is now almost universally measured as the number of connections.

Bibliography

Abbott, J. *Sharing the City: Community Participation in Urban Management.* London: Earthscan Publications, 1996.

Allison, M. C. "Balancing Responsibility for Sanitation." *Social Science and Medicine* 55, no. 9 (2002): 1539–51.

American Society of Civil Engineers. *Existing Sewer Evaluation and Rehabilitation.* Reston, VA: ASCE, 1994.

———. "Report Card for America's Infrastructure." 1998. http://www.asce.org/reportcard (accessed November 23, 2004).

———. "The Grading Process." http://sections.asce.org/colorado/RC/grading.htm (accessed October 18, 2004).

Annis, Sheldon, and Peter Hakim, eds. *Direct to the Poor: Grassroots Development in Latin America.* Boulder, CO, and London: Lynne Rienner Publishers, 1988.

Arnstein, Sherry R. "A Ladder of Citizen Participation." *Journal of the American Institute of Planners* 35, no. 4 (1969): 216–24.

Aycrigg, Maria. "Participation and the World Bank: Success, Constraints, and Responses." *World Bank Social Development Paper* 29 (1998).

Ayee, J., and R. Crook. "Toilet Wars: Urban Sanitation Services and the Politics of Public-Private Partnerships in Ghana." *Institute for Development Studies Working Paper* 213 (2003).

Azevedo-Netto, José M. "Simplified Sewerage System: Technical Aspects." Presentation, Seminario Latino-Americano sobre Saneamento para População de Baixa Renda em Comunidades Rurais e Periurbanas, Recife Palace Hotel, Recife, Pernambuco, Brasil, September 29–October 5, 1988.

———. "Innovative and Low Cost Technologies Utilized in Sewerage." *Pan American Health Organization/World Health Organization-Environmental Health Program Technical Series* 29 (1992).

Bakalian, Alexander, and N. Vijay Jagannathan. "Institutional Aspects of the Condominial Sewer System." *World Bank Infrastructure Notes: Water and Sanitation* SW-6 (August 1991).

Bakalian, Alexander, Albert M. Wright, Richard J. Otis, and José M. de Azevedo Netto. "Simplified Sewerage Meets Demands." *Water Environment and Technology* (1993): 58–62.

———. *Simplified Sewerage: Design Guidelines.* Washington, DC: The World Bank, 1994.

Bauzon, Kenneth E., ed. *Development and Democratization in the Third World: Myths, Hopes and Realities.* Washington, DC: Taylor and Francis, 1992.

Bell, M., and R. Franceys. "Improving Human Welfare through Appropriate Technology: Government Responsibility, Citizen Duty or Customer Choice." *Social Science and Medicine* 40, no. 9 (1995): 1169–79.

Bennett, A. "Causal Inference in Case Studies: From Mill's Methods to Causal Mechanisms." 1999. http://www.georgetown.edu/faculty/bennetta/APSA99.html (accessed November 19, 2004).

Bernard, H. Russell. *Research Methods in Anthropology: Qualitative and Quantitative Approaches.* Thousand Oaks, CA: Sage, 1994.

Birckmayer, J. D., and C. H. Weiss. "Theory-Based Evaluation in Practice: What Do We Learn?" *Evaluation Review* 24, no. 4 (2000): 407–31.

Boschi, Renato Raul. *The Art of Associating: Social Movements, The Middle Class, and Grassroots Politics in Urban Brazil.* New York: Tinker Foundation, 1984.

Bourdieu, Pierre. "The Forms of Capital." In *Handbook of Theory and Research for the Sociology of Education,* edited by John G. Richardson, 241–58. New York: Greenwood Press, 1986.

Briscoe, John, and Harvey A. Garn. "Financing Water Supply and Sanitation under Agenda 21." *Natural Resources Forum* 19, no. 1 (1995): 59–70.

Brown, K., and P. B. Coulter. "Subjective and Objective Measures of Police Service Delivery." *Public Administration Review* 43, no. 1 (1983): 50–58.

Brudney, J. L., and R. E. England. "Urban Policy Making and Subjective Service Evaluations: Are They Compatible?" *Public Administration Review* 42, no. 2 (1982): 127–35.

———. "Toward a Definition of the Co-Production Concept." *Public Administration Review* 43, no. 1 (1983): 59–65.

Bryant, Coralie, and Louise G. White. *Managing Development in the Third World.* Boulder, CO: Westview Press, 1982.

Buso, Alfredo Luiz, Katia Mello, and Marcos Costa Lima. "Integrated Urban Development: The Dike Project in Santos." In *The Challenge of Sustainable Cities: Neoliberalism and Urban Strategies in Developing Countries,* edited by Rod Burgess, Marisa Carmona, and Theo Kolstee. London and New Jersey: Zed Books, 1997.

Cabrera, Ricardo. "Review of 'Rural Water and Sanitation Project' Evaluations in Latin America." CARE International, 1995.

Cairncross, Sandy, and Richard G. Feachem. *Environmental Health Engineering in the Tropics: An Introductory Text*. Chichester, UK: John Wiley & Sons, 1993.

Callon, Michel. "Some Elements of a Sociology of Translation: Domestication of the Scallops and the Fishermen of St. Brieuc Bay." In *Power, Action, and Belief: A New Sociology of Knowledge? (Sociological Review Monograph 32)*, edited by John Law, 196–233. London: Routledge & Kegan Paul, 1986.

Campbell, Tim. *The Quiet Revolution: Decentralization and the Rise of Political Participation in Latin American Cities*. Pittsburgh, PA: University of Pittsburgh Press, 2003.

Carvalho, Jesse M. "Sistema Condominial de Esgoto: A Experiencia da EMBASA no Programa Bahia Azul, Salvador-BA." Paper presented at Seminario Esgoto Condominial de SANEPAR Congresso. Curitiba, Brasil, September 1–2, 2004.

Chambers, Robert. *Whose Reality Counts?: Putting the First Last*. London: Intermediate Technology Publications, 1997.

Chaplin, S. "Cities, Sewers, and Poverty: India's Politics of Sanitation." *Environment and Urbanization* 11, no. 1 (1999): 145–58.

Chelimsky, E., and W. Shadish, eds. *Evaluation for the 21st Century: A Handbook*. Thousand Oaks, CA: Sage, 1997.

Choguill, Marisa B. Guaraldo. "A Ladder of Community Participation for Underdeveloped Countries." *Habitat International* 20, no. 3 (1996): 431–44.

Collier, David, and James Mahoney. "Insights and Pitfalls: Selection Bias in Qualitative Research." *World Politics* 49, no. 1 (1996): 56–91.

Cooke, Bill, and Uma Kothari, eds. *Participation: The New Tyranny?* London and New York: Zed Books, 2001.

Corbitt, Robert. *Standard Handbook of Environmental Engineering*. New York: McGraw-Hill, 1990.

Day, Diane. "Citizen Participation in the Planning Process: An Essentially Contested Concept?," *Journal of Planning Literature* 11, no. 3 (1997): 421–34.

De Vries, Jaap, Micaela Schuster, Paul Procee, and Harry Mengers. "Environmental Management of Small and Medium Sized Cities in Latin America and the Caribbean," Inter-American Development Bank Working Paper, Washington, DC, 2001, http://www.iadb.org/sds/ENV/publication/publication_195_2069_e.htm (accessed October 2, 2005).

Elmendorf, Mary and Patricia Buckles. "Sociocultural Aspects of Water Supply and Excreta Disposal." *World Bank—Appropriate Technology for Water Supply and Sanitation* 5 (1980).

Escobar, Arturo. "Planning." In *The Development Dictionary: A Guide to Knowledge as Power*, edited by Wolfgang Sachs, 132–45. London and New York: Zed Books, 1992.

———. *Encountering Development: The Making and Unmaking of the Third World*. Princeton, NJ: Princeton University Press, 1995.

Esrey, Steven A., James B. Potash, Leslie Roberts, and Clive Shiff. "Quantifying the Health Effects of Water and Sanitation Projects." *World Bank Infrastructure Notes: Water and Sanitation* WS-4 (February 1991).

Esteva, Gustavo, and Madhu Suri Prakash, eds. *Grassroots Post-Modernism: Remaking the Soil of Cultures*. London: Zed Books, 1998.

Fass, S. M. "Water and Poverty: Implications for Water Planning." *Water Resources Research* 29, no. 7 (1993): 1975–81.

Feachem, Richard G. "Community Participation in Appropriate Water Supply and Sanitation Technologies: The Mythology for the Decade." *Proceedings of the Royal Society of London* B209, no. 1174 (July 1980): 15–29.

Feachem, Richard G., Michael McGarry, and Duncan Mara (eds.). *Water, Wastes and Health in Hot Climates*. New York, NY: John Wiley & Sons, Inc., 1977.

Ferguson, James. *The Anti-Politics Machine: "Development," Depoliticization, and Bureaucratic Power in Lesotho*. New York, NY: Cambridge University Press, 1990.

———. *Expectations of Modernity: Myths and Meanings of Urban Life on the Zambian Copperbelt*. Berkeley, CA: University of California Press, 1999.

Fetterman, D. "Empowerment Evaluation: A Response to Patton and Scriven." *Evaluation Practice* 18, no. 3 (1997): 253–66.

Finsterbusch, Kurt, and Warren A. Van Wicklin. "The Contribution of Beneficiary Participation to Development Project Effectiveness." *Public Administration and Development* 7 (1987): 1–23.

Fisher, M. J. "Technology to Fight Poverty and Kick-Start Growth: Helping the Poor to Help Themselves." Paper presented at Stanford University Engineers for a Sustainable World 2004 National Conference. Stanford, CA, October 2, 2004.

Foster, V. *Condominial Water and Sewerage Systems: Costs of Implementation of the Model*. Washington, DC: The World Bank.

Gardner, Katy. "Mixed Messages: Contested 'Development' and the 'Plantation Rehabilitation Project.'" In *Discourses of Development: Anthropological Perspectives*, edited by Grillo and Stirrat. Oxford, UK: Berg, 1997.

Garfinkel, H. *Studies in Ethnomethodology*. New Jersey: Prentice Hall, 1967.

Gay, R. "Neighborhood Associations and Political Change in Rio de Janeiro." *Latin American Research Review* 25, no. 1 (1990): 102–18.

———. *Popular Organization and Democracy in Rio de Janeiro: A Tale of Two Favelas*. Philadelphia, PA: Temple University Press, 1994.

George, A., and A. Bennett. *Case Studies and Theory Development in the Social Sciences*. Cambridge, MA: MIT Press, 2005.

Gerschman, S. "The Role of Social Movements in the Formulation of Health Policy in Brazil." Paper presented at Stanford University Center for Latin American Studies, Stanford, CA, March 3, 1993.

Gerson, Philip R. "Popular Participation in Economic Theory and Practice," *Human Resources Development and Operations Policy Working Paper* 18 (internal working paper). Washington, DC: World Bank, 1993.

Gieryn, T. F. *Cultural Boundaries of Science: Credibility on the Line*. Chicago, IL: University of Chicago Press, 1999.

Glaser, Barney G., and Anselm L. Strauss. *The Discovery of Grounded Theory: Strategies for Qualitative Research*. Chicago, IL: Aldine Pub. Co., 1967.

Goethert, R. "Special Interest Group in Urban Settlements." http://web.mit.edu/sigus/www (accessed October 20, 2005).

Goetz, A. M., and J. Gaventa. "Bringing Citizen Voice and Client Focus into Service Delivery." Working Paper No. 138, Brighton Institute of Development Studies, 2001.

Goodland, Robert, Laura Orlando, and Jeff Anhang, eds. *Toward Sustainable Sanitation*. 2001. http://riles.org (accessed November 23, 2009).

Gorell, Richard A., "Families in Shantytowns in Sao Paulo, Brazil, 1945–1984: The Rural-Urban Connection." Ph.D. dissertation, Lawrence, KS: University of Kansas, 1990.

Grillo, R. D., and R. L. Stirrat, eds. *Discourses of Development: Anthropological Perspectives*. Oxford, UK: Berg, 1997.

Harrison, E. "Big Fish and Small Ponds: Aquaculture Development from the FAO, Rome, to Luapula Province, Zambia." Doctor of Philosophy thesis, University of Sussex, 1995.

Haughton, G. "Environmental Justice and the Sustainable City." In *Earthscan Reader in Sustainable Cities,* edited by D. Satterthwaite. London: Earthscan Publications, 1999.

Healy, Stephen. "Toward a Vocabulary for Speaking of the Engagement of Things into Discourse." *Journal of Environmental Policy and Planning* 7, no. 3 (2005): 239–56.

Heller, L. "Who Really Benefits from Environmental Sanitation Services in the Cities? An Intra-Urban Analysis in Betim, Brazil." *Environment and Urbanization* 11, no. 1 (1999): 133–44.

Hinton, P. R. *Statistics Explained: A Guide for Social Science Students*. London: Routledge, 1995.

Hobart, Mark, ed. *Discourses of Development: Anthropological Perspectives*. London and New York: Routledge, 1993.

Hochstetler, Kathryn. "Democratizing Pressures from Below? Social Movements in the New Brazilian Democracy." In *Democratic Brazil: Actors, Institutions, and Processes*, edited by Peter R. Kingstone and Timothy J. Power, 162–82. Pittsburgh, PA: University of Pittsburgh Press, 2000.

Hoffmann, Birgitte, S. B. Nielsen, M. Elle, S. Gabriel, A. M. Eilersen, M. Henze, and P. S. Mikellsen. "Assessing the Sustainability of Small Wastewater Systems: A Context-Oriented Planning Approach." *Environmental Impact Assessment Review* 20 (2000): 347–57.

Hoffman, Helga. "Poverty and Prosperity in Brazil: What Is Changing?" In *Social Change in Brazil, 1945–1985: The Incomplete Transition*, edited by Edmar L. Bacha and Herbert S. Klein. Albuquerque, NM: University of New Mexico Press, 1989.

Huck, S. W. *Reading Statistics and Research.* New York: Addison Wesley Longman, 2000.
Informant 1, engineering consultant, former city official, and former state official. 1994–1995. Interviews by author. Transcripts. Recife, Brazil.
Informant 2, engineer of a civil engineering company. 1994. Interview by author. Transcript. May 17. Recife, Brazil.
Informant 3, architect, assistant to the president of a Recife sewer agency, former director of a condominial sewer program, and former COMPESA staff member. 1994–1995. Interviews by author. Transcripts. Recife, Brazil.
Informant 4, sociologist, former EMLURB staff member, former director of a condominial sewer program, and former COMPESA staff member. 1994–1995. Interviews by author. Transcripts. Recife, Brazil.
Informant 5, URB director of condominial sewer development. 1994–1995. Interview by author. Transcript. May. Recife, Brazil.
Informant 7, URB sanitation department chief. 1994–1995. Interviews by author. Transcripts. Recife, Brazil.
Informant 8, City of Recife official. 1994–1995. Interview by author. Transcript. Recife, Brazil.
Informant 9, EMLURB engineer and former COMPESA staff member. 1994–1995. Interviews by author. Transcripts. Recife, Brazil.
Informant 10, assistant to the COMPESA financial planning directorate. 1994. Interview by author. Transcript. Recife, Brazil.
Informant 11, COMPESA engineer. 1994. Interview by author. Transcript. Recife, Brazil.
Informant 12, COMPESA engineer, former chief of the COMPESA alternative technology division, and member of COMPESA design review committees. 1994–1995. Interviews by author. Transcripts. Recife, Brazil.
Informant 13, COMPESA engineer. 1994. Interview by author. Transcript. Recife, Brazil.
Informant 15, Secretary of Infrastructure official. 1994–1995. Interview by author. Transcript. Recife, Brazil.
Informant 16, president of a Recife sewer agency. 1994. Interview by author. Transcript. Recife, Brazil.
Informant 17, engineer and professor of the Recife technical school. 1994. Interview by author. Transcript. Recife, Brazil.
Informant 20, URB participation staff member and former COHAB participation staff member. 1994–1995. Interview by author. Transcript. Recife, Brazil.
Informant 22, EMLURB social worker. 1994–1995. Interview by author. Transcript. Recife, Brazil.
Informant 23, EMLURB staff member. 1994–1995. Interview by author. Transcript. Recife, Brazil.
Informant 24, Federal University of Pernambuco professor and former architect for a Recife engineering company. 1994. Interview by author. Transcript. Recife, Brazil.

Informant 29, COMPESA operations and maintenance coordinator. Interview by author. Transcript. December. Recife, Brazil.
Informant 30, engineer and assistant to the president of a Recife sewer agency. Interview by author. Transcript. March 9. Recife, Brazil.
Informant 31, consulting engineer. Interview by author. Transcript. March 3. Recife, Brazil.
Informant 37, COMPESA technical director. Interview by author. Transcript. November 23. Recife, Brazil.
Informant 38, EMLURB condominial sewer intern. 1994–1995. Interview by author. Transcript. Recife, Brazil.
Informant 39, EMLURB condominial sewer intern. 1994–1995. Interview by author. Transcript. Recife, Brazil.
Informant 40, EMLURB condominial sewer staff member. 1994–1995. Interview by author. Transcript. Recife, Brazil.
Informant 41, COMPESA maintenance staff member. 1994–1995. Interview by author. Transcript. Recife, Brazil.
Informant 43, COMPESA billing division staff member. 1994–1995. Interview by author. Transcript. Recife, Brazil.
Informant 44, COMPESA billing division staff member. 1994–1995. Interview by author. Transcript. Recife, Brazil.
Informant 46, URB participation staff member and former COHAB participation staff member. 1994–1995. Interview by author. Transcript. Recife, Brazil.
Informant 51, COMPESA computer information division staff member. 1994–1995. Interview by author. Transcript. Recife, Brazil.
Informant 52, URB participation staff member. 1994–1995. Interview by author. Transcript. Recife, Brazil.
Informant 53, COMPESA maps division staff member. 1994–1995. Interview by author. Transcript. Recife, Brazil.
Informant 54, COMPESA maps division director. 1994–1995. Interview by author. Transcript. Recife, Brazil.
Informant 58, COHAB staff member. 1994–1995. Interview by author. Transcript. Recife, Brazil.
Informant 59, COMPESA division chief. 1994–1995. Interview by author. Transcript. Recife, Brazil.
Informant 62, URB maps division staff member. 1994–1995. Interview by author. Transcript. Recife, Brazil.
Informant 63, URB maps division staff member. 1994–1995. Interview by author. Transcript. Recife, Brazil.
Informant 64, Case R3 community leader and resident. 1994–1995. Interviews by author. Transcripts. Recife, Brazil.
Informant 65, Case R3 community leader and resident. 1994–1995. Interviews by author. Transcripts. Recife, Brazil.
Informant 67, Case R2 community leader. 1994–1995. Interview by author. Transcript. Recife, Brazil.

Informant 68, Case R2 community leader. 1994–1995. Interview by author. Transcript. Recife, Brazil.
Informant 73, Case R1 community leader and resident. 1994–1995. Interviews by author. Transcripts. Recife, Brazil.
Informant 74, Case R1 community leader and resident. 1988. Letter to the Director President of the Secretary of Public Works of Recife (OBRAS). August 22. Recife, Brazil.
Informant 75, CAERN senior civil engineer and sewer construction coordinator. 1994–1995. Interviews by author. Transcripts. Natal, Brazil.
Informant 76, CAERN social worker. 1994–1995. Interviews by author. Transcripts. Natal, Brazil.
Informant 77, CAERN civil engineer. 1994–1995. Interviews by author. Transcripts. Natal, Brazil.
Informant 78, CAERN sewer projects division chief. 1994–1995. Interviews by author. Transcripts. Natal, Brazil.
Informant 79, CAERN planning division chief. 1995. Interview by author. Transcript. Natal, Brazil.
Informant 81, CAERN billing division staff member. 1995. by author. Transcript. Natal, Brazil.
Informant 83, CAERN engineering director. 1995. Interview by author. Transcript. Natal, Brazil.
Informant 84, CAERN maintenance division chief and engineer. 1995. Interview by author. Transcript. Natal, Brazil.
Informant 85, CAERN participation staff member. 1995. Interview by author. Transcript. Natal, Brazil.
Informant 87, CAERN engineer. 1995. Interview by author. Transcript. Natal, Brazil.
Informant 88, CAERN maintenance technician. 1995. Interview by author. Transcript. Natal, Brazil.
Informant 89, CAERN senior maintenance technician. 1995. Interview by author. Transcript. Natal, Brazil.
Informant 90, Federal University of Rio Grande do Norte professor and engineering consultant. 1994–5. Interviews by author. Transcripts. Natal, Brazil.
Informant 91, CAERN staff member. 1995. Interview by author. Transcript. Natal, Brazil.
Informant 92, CAERN participation staff member. 1995. Interview by author. Transcript. Natal, Brazil.
Informant 94, CAERN maintenance technician. 1995. Interview by author. Transcript. Natal, Brazil.
Informant 96, CAERN civil engineer. 1995. Interview by author. Transcript. May 25. Natal, Brazil.
Informant 98, director/president of a Natal sewer agency. 1995. Interview by author. Transcript. Natal, Brazil.
Informant 99, elected official. 1995. Interview by author. Transcript. June 27. Natal, Brazil.

Informant 100, president of an engineering company. 1995. Interview by author. Transcript. March 19. Recife, Brazil.
Informant 101, civil engineer for an engineering company. 1995. Interview by author. Transcript. Recife, Brazil.
Informant 102, civil engineer for an engineering company. 1995. Interview by author. Transcript. Recife, Brazil.
Informant 103, URB infrastructure department engineering manager. 1995. Interview by author. Transcript. Recife, Brazil.
Informant 105, COMPESA operations supervisor. 1995. Interview by author. Transcript. Recife, Brazil.
Informant 106, COMPESA maintenance staff member. Interview by author. Transcript. 1995, Recife, Brazil.
Informant 107, engineering professor and Case R1 resident. 1995. Letter to the Manager of Sewer Services for COMPESA. February 13. Recife, Brazil.
Informant 120, URBANA civil engineer. 1995. Interview by author. Transcript. Natal, Brazil.
Informant 121, CAERN sewer construction division manager. 1995. Interview by author. Transcript. Natal, Brazil.
Informant 122, CAERN staff member. 1995. Interview by author. Transcript. Natal, Brazil.
Informant 123, CAERN civil engineer. 1995. Interview by author. Transcript. Natal, Brazil.
Instituto Brasileiro de Geografia e Estatística, "PNAD (National Household Sample Survey)." 2011. ftp://ftp.ibge.gov.br/Trabalho_e_Rendimento/Pesquisa_Nacional_por_Amostra_de_Domicilios_anual/2011/Sintese_Indicadores/sintese_pnad2011.pdf (accessed October 8, 2012).
———. 2010, http://www.ibge.gov.br/estadosat/perfil.php?sigla=pe (accessed October 8, 2012).
———. 2010, http://www.ibge.gov.br/estadosat/perfil.php?sigla=rn (accessed October 8, 2012).
———. 2010, http://www.ibge.gov.br/english/estatistica/populacao/censo2010/default.shtm (accessed October 8, 2012).
———. 2010, http://www.ibge.gov.br/home/estatistica/populacao/trabalhoerendimento/pnad2005/sintese/tab1_3.pdf (accessed October 8, 2012).
———. "PNAD (National Household Sample Survey)." 2005. http://www.ibge.gov.br/home/estatistica/populacao/trabalhoerendimento/pnad2005/sintesepnad2005.pdf (accessed October 8, 2012).
———. "Brazil 2001." 2001. http://www.IBGE.gov.br/english/presidencia/noticias/12062003indic2002.shtm (accessed October 19, 2005).
———. "Pesquisa Nacional por Amostra de Domicílios (National Household Sample Survey)." 2001. http://www.ibge.gov.br/english/presidencia/noticias/12062003indic2002.shtm (accessed March 29, 2004).
———. "Census Data." 2000. http://www.ibge.gov.br/ (accessed October 19, 2005).

———. "PNAD (National Household Sample Survey)." 1999. http://www.ibge.gov.br/english/estatistica/populacao/trabalhorendimento/pnad99/planotabular/tabbr4_1.shtm (accessedSeptember 19, 2003).

———. "PNAD (National Household Sample Survey)." 1999. http://www.ibge.gov.br/english/estatistica/populacao/trabalhorendimento/pnad99/planotabular/tabbr7_6a.shtm (accessed September 19, 2003).

———. "PNAD (National Household Sample Survey)." 1999. http://www.ibge.gov.br/english/estatistica/populacao/trabalhorendimento/pnad99/sintese/tab7_1_15.shtm (accessed September 19, 2003).

International Organization for Migration. *Migrants Remittances and Development: Myths, Rhetoric and Realities.* 2006.

IRC International Water and Sanitation Centre. "History of Community Management." http://www2.irc.nl/manage/whatisit/history.html (accessed September 13, 2005).

Isham, Jonathan, and Satu Kahkonen. "What Determines the Effectiveness of Community-Based Water Projects: Evidence from Central Java, Indonesia on Demand, Responsiveness, Service Rules, and Social Capital." *Social Capital Initiative Working Paper No. 14.* Washington, DC: The World Bank, 1999.

Isham, Jonathan, Deepa Narayan, and Lant Pritchett. "Does Participation Improve Performance? Establishing Causality with Subjective Data." *World Bank Economic Review* 9, no. 2 (1995): 175–200.

Janssens, J. G., L. Pintelon, A. Cotton, and L. Gelders. "Development of a Framework for the Assessment of Operation and Maintenance (O&M) Performance of Urban Water Supply and Sanitation." *Water Supply* 14, no. 1 (1996): 21–33.

Joshi, Anuradha, and Mick Moore. "Institutionalized Co-Production: Unorthodox Public Service Delivery in Challenging Environments." *Journal of Development Studies* 40, no. 4 (2004): 31–49.

Katzman, Martin T. "Urbanization since 1945," in *Social Change in Brazil, 1945-1985: The Incomplete Transition,* eds. Edmar L. Bacha and Herbert S. Klein. Albuquerque, NM: University of New Mexico Press, 1989.

Kelly, J. M., and D. Swindell. "A Multiple-Indicator Approach to Municipal Service Evaluation: Correlating Performance Measurement and Citizen Satisfaction across Jurisdictions." *Public Administration Review* 62, no. 5 (2002a): 610–21.

———. "Service Quality Variation across Urban Space: First Steps toward a Model of Citizen Satisfaction." *Journal of Urban Affairs* 24, no. 3 (2002b): 271–88.

Khwaja, Asim I. "Is Increasing Community Participation Always a Good Thing?" *Journal of the European Economic Association* 2, no. 2–3 (2004): 427–36.

———. "Can Good Projects Succeed in Bad Communities? Collective Action in Public Good Provision." *John F. Kennedy School of Government Faculty Research Working Papers.* Cambridge, MA: Harvard University, 2002.

Korten, David C. "Community Organization and Rural Development: A Learning Process Approach." *Public Administration Review* 40 (1980): 480–511.

Korten, David C., and Felipe B. Alfonso. *Bureaucracy and the Poor: Closing the Gap*. West Hartford: Kumarian Press, 1983.

Kulipossa, F. P. "Decentralisation and Democracy in Developing Countries: An Overview." *Development in Practice* 14, no. 6 (2004): 768–79.

Latour, B. *Laboratory Life: The Construction of Scientific Facts*. Princeton, NJ: Princeton University Press, 1979.

———. "The Powers of Association." In *Power, Action, and Belief: A New Sociology of Knowledge?*, edited by John Law, 264–80. *Sociological Review Monograph* 32, 264–80. London: Routledge & Kegan Paul, 1986.

———. *Science in Action: How to Follow Scientists and Engineers through Society*. Milton-Keynes UK: Open University Press, 1987.

———. *We Have Never Been Modern*. Cambridge, MA: Harvard University Press, 1993.

———. *Pandora's Hope: Essays on the Reality of Science Studies*. Cambridge, MA: Harvard University Press, 1999.

———. "On Recalling ANT." In *Actor Network Theory and After*, edited by John Law and John Hassard. Oxford: Blackwell Publishers, 1999.

———. *Politics of Nature: How to Bring the Sciences into Democracy*. Cambridge, MA: Harvard University Press, 2004.

———. *Reassembling the Social: An Introduction to Actor-Network-Theory*. Oxford: Oxford University Press, 2005.

Lavalle, A. G., A. Arnab, and P. P. Houtzager. "Beyond Comparative Anecdotalism: Lessons on Civil Society and Participation from Sao Paulo, Brazil." *World Development* 33, no. 6 (2005): 951–64.

Leal S. *Fetiche da Participação Popular: Novas Practicas de Planejamento, Gestao e Governanca Democratica no Recife, Brasil*. Recife, Brazil: Companhia Editora de Pernambuco, 2003.

Lee, Nick, and Paul Stenner. "Who Pays? Can We Pay Them Back?" In *Actor Network Theory and After*, edited by John Law and John Hassard. Oxford: Blackwell Publishers, 1999.

Leeds, Anthony. "Lower-Income Urban Settlement Types: Processes, Structures, Policies." In *The Residential Circumstances of the Urban Poor in Developing Countries*, United Nations Centre for Human Settlements. New York: Praeger Publishers, 1981.

Lemos, M. C., D. Austin, R. Meredith, and R. G. Varady. "Public-Private Partnerships as Catalysts for Community-Based Water Infrastructure Development: The Border Water Works Program in Texas and New Mexico Colonias." *Environment and Planning C: Government and Policy* 20 (2002): 281–95.

Lemos, M. C., and J. W. Looye. "Looking for Sustainability: Environmental Coalitions across the State-Society Divide." *Bulletin of Latin American Research* 22, no. 3 (2003): 350–70.

Levine, C. H. "Citizenship and Service Delivery—The Promise of Co-Production." *Public Administration Review* 44 (1984): 178–87.

Lineberry, R. L. *Equality and Urban Policy: The Distribution of Municipal Services.* Beverly Hills, CA: Sage, 1977.

Lobo, Luiz. "Sistemas Condominiais: A Experiencia na Bolivia." Paper presented at Seminario Esgoto Condominial de SANEPAR Congresso. Curitiba, Brasil, September 1–2, 2004.

Long, N. Introduction to *Battlefields of Knowledge: The Interlocking of Theory and Practice in Social Research and Development*, edited by N. Long and A. Long. London: Routledge, 1992.

Loomis, J. B. *Integrated Public Lands Management: Principles and Applications to National Forests, Parks, Wildlife Refuges, and BLM Lands.* New York: Columbia University Press, 2002.

Mainwaring, Scott. "Grassroots Popular Movements, Identity, and Democratization in Brazil." Working paper no. 84, Helen Kellogg Institute for International Studies, 1986.

———. "Grassroots Popular Movements and the Struggle for Democracy: Nova Iguacu." In *Democratizing Brazil: Problems of Transition and Consolidation*, edited by Alfred Stepan, 168–204. New York and Oxford: Oxford University Press, 1989.

———. *Rethinking Party Systems in the Third Wave of Democratization: The Case of Brazil.* Stanford, CA: Stanford University Press, 1999.

Mara, Duncan. *Low-Cost Urban Sanitation.* Chichester, UK: John Wiley and Sons, 1996.

Mariz, Ricardo. "Tecnologias Alternativas e Integradas para o Saneamento Ambiental." Paper presented at Seminario Esgoto Condominial de SANEPAR Congresso. Curitiba, Brasil, September 1–2, 2004.

Marsden, D. "Indigenous Management: Introduction." In *Anthropology of Organizations*, edited by S. Wright. London, UK: Routledge, 1994.

McGranahan, G., P. Jacobi, J. Songsore, C. Surjadi, and M. Kjellen. *The Citizens at Risk: From Urban Sanitation to Sustainable Cities.* London: Stockholm Environmental Institute and Earthscan Publications, 2001.

McGranahan, G., and D. Satterthwaite. "Environmental Health or Ecological Sustainability? Reconciling the Brown and Green Agendas in Urban Development." In *Sustainable Cities in Developing Countries: Theory and Practice at the Millennium*, edited by C. Pugh. London: Earthscan Publications, 2000.

Mejia, Abel, L. C. Tavares, Alexander Bakalian, and Vijay Jagannathan, "Water and Sanitation Services for the Urban Poor in Brazil: The PROSANEAR Approach," *World Bank Infrastructure Notes-Water and Sanitation* SW9. Washington, DC: World Bank, 1993.

Melo, José Carlos Rodrigues de. *The Experience of Condominial Water and Sewerage Systems in Brazil: Case Studies from Brasília, Salvador, and Parauapebas.* Washington, DC: The World Bank, 2005.

Melo, José Carlos Rodrigues de. *Sistema Condominial de Esgotos: Razões, Teoría, e Prática*. Brasília: Caixa Econômica Federal, 1994.

Melo, José Carlos Rodrigues de. "Sistemas Condominiais de Esgotos." *Engenharia Sanitaria 24*, no. 2 (Abr/Jun, 1985): 237-38. Rio De Janeiro, Brasil.

Menendez, Aurelio. "Access to Basic Infrastructure by the Urban Poor." *Economic Development Institute Policy Seminar Report No. 28*. Washington, DC: The World Bank, 1991.

Meshack, M. V. "Potential and Limitations of Stakeholders' Participation in Community-Based Projects." *International Development Planning Review* 26, no. 1 (2004): 61–82.

Miranda, Ernani Ciriaco de. "Desafios para a Universalização dos Servicos de Esgotamento Sanitario no Brasil: A Visao do Governo Federal." Paper presented at Seminario Esgoto Condominial de SANEPAR Congresso. Curitiba, Brasil, September 1–2, 2004.

Mohr, L. B. "The Impact Profile Approach to Policy Merit: The Case of Research Grants and the University." *Evaluation Review* 23, no. 2 (1999): 212–49.

Mol, Annemarie. "Ontological Politics. A Word and Some Questions." In *Actor Network Theory and After*, edited by John Law and John Hassard. Oxford: Blackwell Publishers, 1999.

———. *The Body Multiple: Multiple Realities in Medicine*. 2003.

Moran, D., and R. Batley. *Literature Review of Non-State Provision of Basic Services*. University of Birmingham Governance Resource Center, 2004: 45–65.

Moser, Caroline O. N. "The Problem of Evaluating Community Participation in Urban Development." In *Evaluating Community Participation in Urban Development Projects,* edited by Caroline O. N. Moser. Working Paper No. 14. London: Development Planning Unit, 1983.

Mosse, David. "People's Knowledge, Participation, and Patronage: Operations and Representations in Rural Development." In *Participation: The New Tyranny?,* edited by Bill Cooke and Uma Kothari. London and New York: Zed Books, 2001.

Nance, Earthea. "Putting Participation in Context: An Evaluation of Urban Sanitation in Brazil." *Dissertation Abstracts International, 65*(04), 2035B. (UMI No 3128354). Ph.D. dissertation, Stanford University, 2004.

———. "Multistakeholder Evaluation of Condominial Sewer Services." *American Journal of Evaluation* 26, no. 4 (2005): 480–500.

Nance, Earthea, and Leonard Ortolano. "Community Participation in Urban Sanitation: Experiences in Northeastern Brazil." *Journal of Planning Education and Research* 26 (2007): 284–300.

Narayan, Deepa. "The Contribution of People's Participation: Evidence from 121 Rural Water Supply Projects." *UNDP-World Bank Water and Sanitation Program (TWUWU) and Social Policy and Resettlement (ENVSP)*. Internal working document, World Bank, 1994.

———. "The Contribution of People's Participation: Evidence from 121 Rural Water Supply Projects." *Environmentally Sustainable Development Occasional Paper Series No. 1*. Washington, DC: The World Bank, 1995.

National Council on Public Works Improvement. "Report Card on the Nation's Public Works." 1998. http://www.asce.org/reportcard (accessed November 23, 2004).

Nazareth, Pery. "Sistemas Condominiais de Esgoto: Estudo Comparado de Experiencias Relevantes e Aspectos Criticos ao Emprego do Modelo Condominial." Paper presented at Seminario Esgoto Condominial de SANEPAR Congresso. Curitiba, Brasil, September 1–2, 2004.

Neto, Cicero Onofre de Andrade. "Modelo Condominial de Esgotamento Sanitário: Conceituação nos Aspetos Tecnico e Social." Paper presented at Seminario Esgoto Condominial de SANEPAR Congresso. Curitiba, Brasil, September 1–2, 2004.

Neto, Cicero Onofre de Andrade, and Aldo da Fonseca Tinoco Filho. "Sistema Condominial de Esgotos de Rocas/Santos Reis, Análise Crítica Mediante Pesquisa de Acompanhamento." Thirteenth Congresso Brasileiro de Engenharia Sanitária e Ambiental, Maceio, CAERN, August 18–23, 1985.

Neto, Cicero Onofre de Andrade, Hercilia Coelho de Medeiros, and José Carlos Rodrigues de Melo. "Currais Novos-Uma Solução de Esgotos com as Menores Perdas." Twelfth Congresso Brasileiro de Engenharia Sanitária e Ambiental, Balneário Camboriú, Santa Catarina, CAERN, 20–25, 1983.

Oakley, P., et al. *Projects with People: The Practice of Participation in Rural Development*. Geneva: International Labour Organization, 1991.

Ostrom, Elinor. "The Need for Multiple Indicators in Measuring the Output of Public Agencies." *Policy Studies Journal* 2, no. 1 (1973): 85–91.

———. *Crafting Institutions for Self-Governing Irrigation Systems*. San Francisco, CA: ICS Press, 1992.

———. "Crossing the Great Divide: Co-Production, Synergy, and Development." *World Development* 24, no. 6 (1996): 1073–88.

Ostrom, Elinor, Roger B. Parks, and Gordon Whitaker. *Patterns of Metropolitan Policing*. Cambridge, MA: Ballinger, 1978.

Ostrom, Elinor, Larry Schroeder, and Susan Wynne. *Institutional Incentives and Sustainable Development: Infrastructure Policies in Perspective*. Boulder, CO: Westview Press, 1993.

Pan American Health Organization (PAHO). "Country Health Profile-Brazil." *Health in the Americas*. 1998. http://www.paho.org/english/sha/prflbra.htm (accessed March 29, 2004).

———. "Special Program for Health Analysis Linear Interpolation Based on UN Data: World Urbanization Prospects, the 1999 Revision." 1999. http://www.paho.org (accessed March 2004).

Parfitt, Trevor. *The End of Development*. London: Pluto Press, 2002.

———. "The Ambiguity of Participation: A Qualified Defense of Participatory Development." *Third World Quarterly* 25, no. 3 (2004): 537–56.

Parks, R. B. "Linking Objective and Subjective Measures of Performance." *Public Administration Review* 44, no. 2 (1984): 118–27.

Parks, Roger, Paula Baker, Larry Kiser, Ronald Oakerson, Elinor Ostrom, Vincent Ostrom, Stephen Percy, Martha Vandivort, Gordon Whitaker, and Rick Wilson. "Co-Production of Public Services." In *Analyzing Urban Service Distributions,* edited by Richard C. Rich, 185–99. Lexington, MA: Lexington Books, 1982.

Parlatore, Antonio Carlos. "Privatization of the Water Utility Sector in Brazil." http://www.bndes.gov.br/english/studies/ensa/0–8.pdf (accessed 2003).

Patton, Michael Quinn. *Qualitative Research and Evaluation Methods.* Thousand Oaks, CA: Sage Publications, 2002.

Paul, Samuel. "Community Participation in Development Projects: The World Bank Experience." *World Bank Discussion Paper No. 6.* Washington, DC: The World Bank, 1987.

Pearce, J. "Collective Action or Public Participation: Complementary or Contradictory Democratisation Strategies in Latin America?" *Bulletin of Latin American Research* 23, no. 4 (2004): 483–504.

Peet, Richard, and Elaine Hartwick. *Theories of Development.* New York: The Guilford Press, 1999.

Percy, S. L. "Citizen Participation in the Co-Production of Urban Services." *Urban Affairs Review* 19, no. 4 (1984):431–46.

———. "In Defense of Citizen Evaluations as Performance Measures." *Urban Affairs Quarterly* 22, no. 1 (1986): 66–83.

Perlman, Janice. *The Myth of Marginality: Urban Politics and Poverty in Rio de Janeiro.* Berkeley: University of California Press, 1976.

Pickering, Andrew. *The Mangle of Practice: Time, Agency, and Science.* Chicago: University of Chicago Press, 1995.

Pickford, John. *Low-Cost Sanitation: A Survey of Practical Experience.* London: Intermediate Technology Publications, 1995.

Pigg, S. L. "Constructing Social Categories through Place: Social Representation and Development in Nepal." *Comparative Studies in Society and History* 34, no. 3 (1992): 491–513.

Populstat, 1999/2003,www.library.uu.nl/wesp/populstat/Americas/brazilp.htm (accessed 2005).

———. 1999/2003,www.library.uu.nl/wesp/populstat/Americas/brazilc.htm (accessed 2005).

———. 1999/2006, http://www.populstat.info/ (accessed 2006).

Power, Timothy J., and J. Timmons Roberts. "A New Brazil? The Changing Sociodemographic Context of Brazilian Democracy," in *Democratic Brazil: Actors, Institutions, and Processes,* eds. Peter R. Kingstone and Timothy J. Power. Pittsburgh, PA: University of Pittsburgh Press, 2000: 248.

Preston, P. W. *Discourses of Development: State, Market and Polity in the Analysis of Complex Change.* Aldershot, UK: Avebury, 1994.

Pritchett, L., and M. Woolcock. "Solutions when *the* Solution Is the Problem: Arraying the Disarray in Development." *World Development* 32, no. 2 (2004): 191–212.

Prokopy, Linda S. "The Relationship between Participation and Project Outcomes: A Study of Rural Drinking Water Projects in India." Ph.D. dissertation, University of North Carolina, 2002.

———. "The Relationship between Participation and Project Outcomes: Evidence from Rural Water Supply Projects in India." *World Development* 33, no. 11 (2005): 1801–19.

Pugh, C., ed. *Sustainable Cities in Developing Countries: Theory and Practice at the Millennium.* London: Earthscan Publications, 2000.

Ragin, Charles C. "Turning the Tables: How Case-Oriented Research Challenges Variable-Oriented Research." *Comparative Social Research* 16 (1997): 27–42.

———. *Fuzzy-Set Social Science.* Chicago: University of Chicago Press, 2000.

Rahnema, Majid, and Victoria Bawtreea, eds. *The Postdevelopment Reader.* London: Zed Books, 1997.

Reader, N.F., G. Tremey, A. Kempe, P. Friis, and M. Garcia-Poveda. "Performance Indicators." *Water Supply* 1(2/3) (1983): SS21-1–SS21-4.

Rich, R. C. "Municipal Service and the Interaction of the Voluntary and Governmental Sectors." *Administration and Society* 13, no. 1 (1981): 59–76.

Rissoli, Cezar. "Sistema Condominial e Universalização dos Servicos de Saneamento no Distrito Federal." Paper presented at Seminario Esgoto Condominial de SANEPAR Congresso. Curitiba, Brasil, September 1–2, 2004.

Rosentraub, M. S., and L. Thompson. "The Use of Surveys of Satisfaction for Evaluations." *Policy Studies Journal* 9, no. 7 (1981): 990–99.

Roth, W. M., J. Riecken, L. Pozzer-Ardenghi, R. McMillan, B. Storr, D. Tait, G. Bradshaw, and T. P. Penner. "Those Who Get Hurt Aren't Always Being Heard: Scientist-Resident Interactions over Community Water." *Science, Technology, and Human Values* 29, no. 2 (2004): 153–83.

Sachs, Wolfgang, ed. *The Development Dictionary: A Guide to Knowledge as Power.* London, and New York: Zed Books Ltd, 1992.

Samuels, David. "Reinventing Local Government? Municipalities and Intergovernmental Relations in Democratic Brazil." In *Democratic Brazil: Actors, Institutions, and Processes,* edited by Peter R. Kingstone and Timothy J. Power. Pittsburgh, PA: University of Pittsburgh Press, 2000.

Sandercock, L. "Out of the Closet: The Importance of Stories and Storytelling in Planning Practice." In *Dialogues in Urban and Regional Planning 1,* edited by B. Stiftel and V. Watson. New York: Routledge, 2004.

Santos, Carlos Alberto dos, and Adejalmo Figueiredo Gazen. "Estudo Comparativo Entre Redes Coletoras de Esgotos do Tipo Convencional e Não Convencional." Convenio ASFAMAS-PVC e ABIVINILA, Artigo Técnico, September 1987.

Sara, Jennifer, and Travis Katz. *Making Rural Water Supply Sustainable: Report on the Impact of Project Rules*. UNDP-World Bank Water and Sanitation Program, 1997.

Sauer, Sergio. "The World Bank and Land Reform in Brazil, Part II," *Land Research Action Network* 2003. http://www.landaction.org/display.php?article=134 (accessed October 2, 2005).

Schalock, R. L. *Outcome-Based Evaluation.* New York: Kluwer Academic/Plenum, 2001.

Schubeler, Peter. "Participative Strategies for Improving Urban Infrastructure and Services in Developing Countries." Paper presented at Workshop for Architecture and Planning, Ltd., UNCHS Habitat, Nairobi, Kenya, 1995.

Scott, James. *Seeing Like a State: How Certain Schemes to Improve the Human Condition Have Failed.* Binghamton, NY: Yale University Press, 1999.

Seddon. D. "Anthropology and Appraisal: The Preparation of Two IFAD Pastoral Development Projects in Niger and Mali." In *Practising Development*, edited by J. Pottier. London, UK: Routledge, 1993.

Silva, Ricardo Toledo. "Urban Reconstruction and Institutional Reshaping in Brazil." In *The Challenge of Sustainable Cities: Neoliberalism and Urban Strategies in Developing Countries*, edited by Rod Burgess, Marisa Carmona, and Theo Kolstee. London and New Jersey: Zed Books, 1997.

Sinnatamby, Gehan S. "Low Cost Sanitation Systems for Urban Peripheral Areas in Northeast Brazil." Ph.D. dissertation, The University of Leeds, England, 1983.

———. "Low Cost Sanitation." In *The Poor Die Young: Housing and Health in Third World Cities*, edited by Sandy Cairncross, Jorge E. Hardoy, and David Satterthwaite, 127–57. London: Earthscan Publications Ltd., 1990.

Soares, Luiz Carlos Rangel, ed., "Regional Report on the Evaluation 2000 in the Region of the Americas: Water Supply and Sanitation, Current Status and Prospects" (Washington, DC: Pan American Health Organization and World Health Organization, 2001), 16–17.

Solo, Tova Maria, Eduardo Perez, and Steven Joyce. "Constraints in Providing Water and Sanitation Services to the Urban Poor." *Water Sanitation and Hygiene Report 85*. Washington, DC: U.S. Agency for International Development, 1993.

Stepan, A. *Democratizing Brazil: Problems of Transition and Consolidation.* New York and Oxford: Oxford University Press, 1989.

Stipak, B. "Citizen Satisfaction with Urban Services: Potential Misuse as a Performance Indicator." *Public Administration Review* 39, no. 1 (1979): 46–52.

Suchman, L. *Plans and Situated Actions: The Problem of Human-Machine Communication.* Cambridge, UK: Cambridge University Press, 1987.

Sundeen, R. A. 1985. "Co-Production and Communities—Implications for Local Administrators" *Administration and Society* 16, no. 4 (1985): 387–402.

Swyngedouw, E., and N. C. Heynen. "Urban Political Ecology, Justice, and the Politics of Scale." *Antipode* 35, no. 5 (2003): 898–918.

Taylor, Harold. "Insights into Participation from Critical Management and Labour Process Perspectives." In *Participation: The New Tyranny?*, edited by Bill Cooke and Uma Kothari. London and New York: Zed Books, 2001.

Tendler, Judith. *Good Government in the Tropics*. Baltimore, MD: Johns Hopkins University Press, 1998.

Thoreau, Henry David. *Walden, or, Life in the Woods*. 1854.

Tolosa, H. C. "Causes of Urban Poverty in Brazil." *World Development* 6, no. 9/10 (1978): 1087–1101.

United Kingdom Office of Water. "Level of Service Indicators." 1998. http://www.ofwat.gov.uk/aptrix/ofwat/publish.nsf/Content/losindicators (accessed November 23, 2004).

United Nations Development Program. "Clean Water and Sanitation for the Poor." 2003. http://www.undp.org/dpa/publications/FSwater120303E.pdf (accessed January 12, 2005).

United Nations Millennium Project. *Investing in Development: A Practical Plan to Achieve the Millennium Development Goals*. New York: United Nations Development Program, 2005.

United Nations Population Division of the Department of Economic and Social Affairs. *World Urbanization Prospects: The 2001 Revision*. 2002. http://www.un.org/esa/population/publications/wup2001/WUP2001report.htm (accessed September 12, 2005).

United States Environmental Protection Agency. *Sewer System Evaluation, Rehabilitation, and New Construction: A Manual of Practice*. No. EPA-600/2-77-017d. Cincinnati, OH: 1977.

———. *Sewer System Infrastructure Analysis and Rehabilitation*. No. EPA/625/6-91/030. Cincinnati, OH: 1991.

———. *Decision-Support Tools for Predicting the Performance of Water Distribution and Wastewater Collection Systems*. Cincinnati, OH: 2002.

Van Ryzin, G. G. "Expectations, Performance, and Citizen Satisfaction with Urban Services." *Journal of Policy Analysis and Management* 23, no. 3 (2004): 433–48.

Vargas-Ramirez, Miguel, and Teresa Cristina Lampoglia. "Scaling-up Using Condominial Technology." *Waterlines* 25, no. 2 (2006).

Verran, Helen. *Science and an African Logic*. Chicago and London: The University of Chicago Press, 2001.

Vines, Marcus, Bob Reed, and John Pickford. "Reduced Cost Sewerage for Developing Countries." Water, Engineering, and Development Centre. Overseas Development Administration, 1990.

Wade, R. "The Management of Irrigation Systems: How to Evoke Trust and Avoid the Prisoners' Dilemma." *World Development* 16, no. 4 (1988): 489–500.

Washington, Rosier, and Goodall. *Echoes from the Poisoned Well: Global Memories of Environmental Injustice*. Lanham, MD: Lexington Books, 2006.

Watson, Gabrielle. *Good Sewers Cheap?: Agency-Customer Interactions in Low-Cost Urban Sanitation in Brazil.* World Bank Water and Sanitation Division. Washington, DC: The World Bank, 1995.

———. "Water and Sanitation in Sao Paulo, Brazil: Successful Strategies for Service Provision in Low-Income Communities." Master's thesis, Cambridge, MA: Massachusetts Institute of Technology, 1992.

Watson, Gabrielle, and N. Vijay Jagannathan. "Participation in Water and Sanitation." *Environment Department Papers: Participation Series*, Paper No. ENV–002. Washington, DC: The World Bank, 1995.

Weiss, Linda. *The Myth of the Powerless State*. Ithaca, NY: Cornell University Press, 1998.

Whitaker, Gordon P. "Coproduction: Citizen Participation in Service Delivery." *Public Administration Review* 40, no. 3 (1980): 240–46.

Wikimapia, http://www.wikimapia.org/1436913/Natal (accessed October 8, 2012).

———. http://www.wikimapia.org/79507/Recife (accessed October 8, 2012).

World Bank. *Benchmarking Water and Sanitation Utilities: Network of Core Indicator Values*. 2004. http://www.worldbank.org/html/fpd/water/topics/bench/bench_network_inddef_ac.html (accessed October 18, 2004).

———. *Project Appraisal Document for the Recife Urban Upgrading Project.* Report No. 23331-BR. Washington, DC: The World Bank, 2003.

———. *World Development Report 1992: Development and the Environment.* Washington, DC: Oxford University Press, 1992.

———. *World Development Report 1994: Infrastructure for Development.* Washington, DC: Oxford University Press, 1994.

———. *World Development Report 2004: Making Services Work for Poor People.* Washington, DC: Oxford University Press, 2004.

———. *Latin American and Caribbean Seminar on Water and Sanitation for Low-Income Groups.* Report, Recife, Brazil, September 29–October 5, 1988. World Bank Water and Sanitation Division, 1989.

World Health Organization. *Global Water Supply and Sanitation Assessment 2000 Report.* 2000. http://www.who.int/docstore/water_sanitation_health/Globassessment/Global1.htm#1.1 (accessed March 29, 2004).

Wright, Albert M. "Toward a Strategic Sanitation Approach: Improving the Sustainability of Urban Sanitation in Developing Countries." In *UNDP-World Bank Water and Sanitation Program,* internal working document. Washington, DC: The World Bank, 1997.

Wright, Albert M., and Alexander E. Bakalian. "Intermediate Sanitation: Cost Efficient Sewerage." *Water and Sanitation No. SW-4.* World Bank Infrastructure Notes, July 1990.

Yepes, G. *Water and Sanitation Utilities: Operational Indicators.* Washington, DC: The World Bank, 1993.

Yi-chong, Xu, and Patrick Weller. *Inside the World Bank: Exploding the Myth of the Monolithic Bank.* New York: Palgrave MacMillian, 2009.

Yin, Robert K. *Case Study Research: Design and Methods*. Thousand Oaks, CA: Sage Publications, 1994.

Index

About the Author

Earthea Nance is an assistant professor in the Department of Planning and Urban Studies at the University of New Orleans. Her research interests are environmental hazards, urban infrastructure, and community participation in complex settings such as developing countries, vulnerable communities, high-hazard areas, and post-disaster settings. Dr. Nance earned an interdisciplinary PhD from Stanford University with a focus on environmental planning and management, Latin American studies, and anthropology. She also holds BS and MS degrees in civil and environmental engineering from the University of California-Davis, and she is a board-licensed civil engineer with fifteen years of professional practice. She previously taught at Virginia Tech and Massachusetts Institute of Technology.

www.ingramcontent.com/pod-product-compliance
Ingram Content Group UK Ltd.
Pitfield, Milton Keynes, MK11 3LW, UK
UKHW041629031026
15587UKWH00001B/172

9 780739 126813